Resources for People

with

Disabilities and Chronic Conditions

Resources for Rehabilitation
Lexington, Massachusetts

Resources for Rehabilitation
33 Bedford Street, Suite 19A
Lexington, Massachusetts 02173
(617) 862-6455

ISBN 0-929718-06-2

Resources for Rehabilitation is a nonprofit organization dedicated to providing training and information to professionals and the public about the needs of individuals with disabilities and the resources available to meet those needs.

Library of Congress Cataloging-in-Publication Data

Resources for People with Disabilities and Chronic Conditions

    Includes bibliographical references
    ISBN 0-929718-06-2
1. Handicapped--Rehabilitation--United States--Directories.
2. Handicapped--Services for--United States--Directories.
3. Chronically ill--Rehabilitation--United States--Directories.
4. Chronically ill--Services for--United States--Directories.
I. Resources for Rehabilitation (Organization)
HV1559.U6R47   1991
362.1'0425--dc20   91-11894
                                                CIP

TABLE OF CONTENTS

HOW TO USE THIS BOOK

The services available for people with disabilities and chronic conditions have increased in recent years to meet the needs of this growing population. The vast array of services and the eligibility criteria for these services may be confusing to individuals and service providers alike. Furthermore, many individuals and service providers are unaware of these services.

This book is designed to help individuals with disabilities and chronic conditions, their family members, and service providers find services and products that contribute to achieving the maximum level of independence possible. It provides information on a wide variety of organizations, publications, and assistive devices. Because individuals have different lifestyles, needs, and degrees of impairment, this book is organized so that individuals may select the services and devices that are most appropriate to their specific needs.

Beginning with Chapter 5, each chapter has introductory material describing causes and effects of the condition or impairment; special information concerning the needs of children and elders, when appropriate; psychological aspects; information on professional service providers and where to find services; assistive devices; major organizations serving people with the condition or disability; and publications and tapes. Listings of organizations, publications and tapes, and assistive devices are alphabetical within sections. Books produced by commercial publishers are available at bookstores and libraries. Publications produced by a service agency are available directly from the agency; therefore, the address and phone number are included for these organizations. All of the material is up-to-date and prices were accurate as of the time of publication. All prices are quoted in U.S. dollars unless otherwise noted.

This volume is updated on a regular basis. To suggest additional information that should be included, write to:

Resources for Rehabilitation
33 Bedford Street, Suite 19A
Lexington, MA 02173

LIVING WITH A DISABILITY OR CHRONIC CONDITION

The number of individuals who live with a disability or chronic condition constitutes a significant proportion of the population. Although the exact number of individuals is not known, estimates commonly cited by government agencies range from 36 million (National Council on Disability: 1986, 3) to 43 million (Americans with Disabilities Act: 1990). Despite the lack of concrete data concerning the number of individuals with a disability or chronic condition, few would dispute that the population is growing.

Several factors contribute to the growth of this population. Advances in medical technology have increased the survival rates of individuals who have experienced severe trauma and babies who are born with diseases that formerly were life-threatening. Similarly, advances in technology have enabled the general population to live longer. An increase in the prevalence of disabilities and chronic conditions has accompanied this increased longevity.

A wide variety of services exists for this population in both the private and public sectors. Federal legislation has mandated a variety of programs that provide rehabilitation services and independent living services. Such programs exist at the state, regional, and local levels. Special programs and services are available at hospitals, libraries, senior centers, independent living centers, and in educational institutions at all levels, from preschool through postsecondary.

Although the services that exist are both numerous and varied, it is commonplace to discover that people who need these services have not received information about them or about the implications of their own condition. Individuals interviewed by William Roth (1981) repeatedly made this point. For example, one individual who was paralyzed said the following about his hospital stay:

> I hardly ever saw or talked with my doctor. An aide used to come by and check me. I think it would have been a lot more helpful for me to talk to the doctor and have him explain all the aspects of my disability and how I could function in my daily life with it. Maybe the doctors didn't know about independent living. But even if they didn't, they should have tried to get me off the catheter and give a lot of counseling to me and my family.

> ... They should have classes for people who are disabled to inform them about their disability and what it means....I probably learned more from other people in wheelchairs than I did from any of the doctors... (1981, pp. 42-43)

Researchers have found that physicians often lack knowledge about rehabilitation services or have a negative attitude toward rehabilitation. Greenblatt (1989) found that ophthalmologists are themselves unaware of many of the services that exist to help people who are visually impaired or blind. Her study of people who had recently been diagnosed with irreversible vision loss found that these individuals are often given a diagnosis with no explanation of the available services or devices that would have enabled them to function independently and to continue working.

Researchers in the field of aphasia noted:

> ...many physicians dismiss aphasia rehabilitation as an irrelevant endeavor...As the 20th century progressed, however, physicians became less involved with aphasia rehabilitation and seemed to adopt the pessimistic attitude of hopelessness" (Albert and Helm-Esta-brooks: 1988, p. 1206)

A negative attitude on the part of some physicians and inadequate information about rehabilitation leave people with disabilities and chronic conditions in a position where they are marginal to both the fields of medicine and rehabilitation. Physicians, who are attuned more to the needs of patients with acute conditions than those with chronic conditions, in essence often write off many of these patients. Rehabilitation professionals are not aware of these patients and therefore are unable to provide services to them. In many instances, these patients never receive rehabilitation services or else years elapse before they do.

RESPONSES TO DISABILITY AND CHRONIC CONDITIONS

The diagnosis of a disability or chronic condition changes a person's life dramatically. To many members of society, people with physical impairments bear a stigma; their social status has decreased and they become the objects of others' curiosity. People with disabilities are aware of the way in which society views them. As a result, some people try to "pass" or to hide their disabilities. Many individuals who experience their first physical impairment in later life once held the same stereotypes that they now fear will be applied to them.

It is normal for people who have recently learned that they have a disability or chronic condition to go through a series of emotions including depression, denial, bargaining, anger, and acceptance. These reactions are similar to those that occur after other losses, such as the death of a loved one. Not every individual experiences all of these reactions. Some people may be chronically depressed; some may deny the permanency or severity of their loss; others may accept the loss and move on to acceptance of rehabilitation services and adaptive aids or devices.

Knowledge of the person's previous reactions to stressful situations may provide insight into his or her responses to a disability or chronic condition. It is common to rely on coping mechanisms that have been developed over a course of a lifetime. Religious faith, family, and friends may help some individuals to face disability and cope with it in a positive manner.

An individual's reactions may be shaped by the severity of the disability or condition and whether it occurs suddenly or gradually. When the onset of disability is gradual and early intervention measures are taken, the individual may be motivated to learn new ways of accomplishing ordinary tasks. In addition, the individual may be better able to handle depression; may retain a positive self-image; and strive to be independent. Both the individual and family members have time to plan for necessary changes, although anxiety over the future course of the condition may be severe.

When a disability or chronic condition has a sudden onset, the individual may be in a state of shock. Depression, the most common response to loss, often follows shock. Both shock and depression are normal precedents to emotional recovery. Depression is not always recognized, because it may be masked by weakness, apathy, irritability, and passivity (Hollander: 1982, 25). Denial of the presence of the disability is also a common reaction. Service providers and family members must not encourage the belief that the condition will be reversed. Individuals must fully accept their condition before emotional recovery can occur. Individuals who deny their conditions should be referred for counseling; otherwise it is unlikely that rehabilitation will be effective.

It is especially difficult for people to cope with those chronic conditions that fluctuate in their severity and impact. Conditions such as multiple sclerosis and diabetes can leave people relatively free of symptoms for a period of time and then cause devastating problems, such as loss of vision. Adjusting to the current situation is difficult enough; add to this the fear that the condition may worsen and it is easy to understand why people in these circumstances have great emotional burdens.

Brooks and Matson (1987) have described the broad array of coping mechanisms and skills that individuals with multiple sclerosis must develop in order to feel that they have a sense of control over their condition and their lives. They must make decisions about medications and treatment; search for information about their disease; adapt their environment to accommodate their current situation; and take measures to relieve anxiety. All of these factors affect employment, family life, and relationships outside the family.

The knowledge that there are services available to help cope with what may at first seem overwhelming can make the difference in maintaining the ability to continue functioning independently. Learning about the various techniques and devices that are constantly being improved by technology may prove to be the factor that enables individuals to come to grips with the new dimension of their lives.

The roles of professional service providers may be crucial in shaping individuals' responses to a disability or a chronic condition. Professionals can help people with disabilities to continue functioning in socially productive roles and to avoid the feeling that they need to "pass." Combating negative attitudes among professionals toward people with disabilities is an essential first step in serving this growing population.

WHERE TO FIND LOCAL SERVICES

A good place to start the search for services is the information and referral office of the local United Way. State and municipal offices established to serve people with disabilities are other sources of referrals. Other sources of information are local directories of service agencies available in the reference collection of many public libraries. Libraries themselves often have special programs for people with disabilities, and some have special needs centers or special reading equipment for people with visual impairments.

Rehabilitation agencies, described below, are a major source of assistance for people with disabilities and chronic conditions. Some departments of rehabilitation, human or health services, and education may provide respite care to families of individuals with disabilities. Respite care is temporary help designed to relieve caretakers of the need to be "on call" for 24 hours a day. It relieves the caretaker's emotional burden and allows time to tend to personal needs.

Veterans are eligible for special benefits and rehabilitation services. In the United States, the Department of Veterans Affairs (VA) has established a number of special services, including the provision of prosthetics for veterans with service related disabilities. Visual Impairment Services Teams (VIST) help veterans with vision problems. The VA will specially adapt the homes of disabled veterans. A booklet describing all of the benefits and rights of veterans, "Federal Benefits for Veterans and Dependents," is available for $2.75 from the Superintendent of Documents, U.S. Government Printing Office, Washington DC 20402.

REHABILITATION

The rehabilitation process helps individuals who have irreversible impairments or chronic conditions to continue functioning in society. Rehabilitation is appropriate when medical and surgical interventions are incapable of restoring the individual's functioning to normal. Rehabilitation services may include any or all of the following:

- rehabilitation counseling
- job placement
- provision of adaptive equipment, prostheses, and medical supplies
- vocational training to remain in one's current position or to learn a new skill
- adapting the home or work environment
- training in activities of daily living and homemaking
- transportation services

Rehabilitation services are provided by both public and private agencies. In the United States, each state is required by law to have a public agency that is responsible for providing vocational rehabilitation services. In about half of the states, there are separate agencies to serve people who are visually impaired or blind. In the remaining states, services for people who are visually impaired or blind are provided within the general vocational rehabilitation agency. Many states offer special rehabilitation services for children and elders. The federal government provides financial support for rehabilitation services and sets standards for service delivery, as required by the Rehabilitation Act of 1973 and its amendments (see Chapter 2, "Laws that Affect People with Disabilities") and administered by the Rehabilitation Services Administration.

Some rehabilitation professionals provide services independently on a fee-for-service basis. (Rehabilitation counselors are certified by the Commission on Rehabilitation Counselor Certification, listed in "ORGANIZATIONS" section below.) Rehabilitation services are offered in group settings, in residential settings, or at home.

There is no one rehabilitation plan that will work for all individuals. Individuals must work jointly with rehabilitation counselors to set their goals and establish an appropriate rehabilitation plan to meet those goals. In fact, the federal government requires that individuals sign an Individual Written Rehabilitation Plan that indicates they approve of the rehabilitation strategy developed jointly with counselors in state rehabilitation agencies. It is also important to involve family members in the rehabilitation process so that they will support, not undermine, the person's attempts to remain independent.

The Client Assistance Program is a federally mandated program that requires states to provide information to all clients and potential clients about the benefits available under the Rehabilitation Act (see Chapter 2, "Laws that Affect People with Disabilities") and to assist clients in obtaining these benefits.

Individuals with severe disabilities often require assistance with personal care, transportation, and special equipment. Independent living programs enable people with disabilities to continue functioning within the community with a minimal amount of assistance. A crucial element of the independent living movement is that consumers have control over the types of services provided. For some, this means living at home, with or without attendant care, and maintaining employment. Attendants assist people with disabilities in activities such as bathing, grooming, dressing, food preparation, and household tasks. Provisions of both Social Security and Medicaid laws have been used to finance the services of attendants. People with disabilities or chronic conditions may opt to live in group residences, where individuals live under supervision but maintain a degree of responsibility for their own care and maintenance. Independent living programs or centers are sometimes administered by rehabilitation agencies and sometimes are free-standing organizations administered by individuals with disabilities themselves.

Ideally, the approach to medical treatment and rehabilitation planning should be carried out jointly by health professionals and rehabilitation professionals. Because the medical profession is oriented toward cure rather than rehabilitation, such a collaborative approach is often a difficult goal to attain.

SELF-HELP GROUPS

Self-help groups enable individuals with similar problems or conditions to discuss their problems and offer mutual assistance. Self-help groups offer a number of benefits to participants, including learning to develop coping strategies; acquiring a sense of control over one's life; combating isolation and alienation; and developing information networks. In addition, members of self-help groups often express a sense of increased self-esteem, because they have offered help to other members of the group.

Self-help group members often believe that their peers are more understanding and patient than professional counselors, health care providers, or even family members, because they have had similar experiences. The person who needs help may feel weak or incompetent, no matter what his or her profession or background. Receiving help from a peer tends to minimize these feelings.

Professional service providers are ideally suited to identify and bring together individuals with common problems, and they often are able to offer a site where meetings may be held. However, professionals must understand the new role that they play in helping to create a self-help group. Madara (no date) recommends that professionals assume the role of consultants, providing advice and counsel but not assuming any responsibility for leadership, decision making, or group tasks. A professional who is the catalyst for the formation of a group must disengage from this initial role to allow the group to develop autonomously. Since professionals often tend to encourage dependent client relationships, they must guard against this type of relationship if a group is to offer true mutual support.

Identifying a group facilitator or coordinator is the first step in developing a self-help group for individuals with disabilities and chronic conditions. One method is to identify someone who has had group experience. Former patients or clients who have had experience in coping with disabilities are likely candidates for starting a group. Another method is to identify an organized, articulate person who has experienced a disability and has some background in a club or other organization. Announcements in publications, at meetings, and on hospital and agency bulletin boards are also good recruitment techniques. Once the group is established, it is up to the members to decide how frequently to meet; the types of discussions or programs to have; and how to recruit members.

CONCLUSION

Rehabilitation, independent living programs, and self-help groups are some of the options available to help individuals with disabilities and chronic conditions. When these local services are used in conjunction with the resources described in this book, people with disabilities and chronic conditions may overcome depression and function to the maximum level of independence possible. The ability to function independently will have great consequences on the individual's self-esteem, on relationships with family members and significant others, and on employment.

References

Albert, Martin and Nancy Helm-Estabrooks
1988 "Diagnosis and Treatment of Aphasia, Part II" JAMA 259(Feb. 26):8: 1205-1210

Americans with Disabilities Act
1990 Public Law 101-336

Brooks, Nancy A. and Ronald R. Matson
1987 "Managing Multiple Sclerosis" Volume 6, pp. 73-106 in Julius A. Roth and Peter Conrad (eds.) Research in the Sociology of Health Care Greenwich, CT: JAI Press Inc.

Greenblatt, Susan L.
1989 "The Need for Coordinated Care" pp. 25-38 in Susan L. Greenblatt, (ed.) Providing Services for People with Vision Loss: A Multidisciplinary Perspective Lexington, MA: Resources for Rehabilitation

Hollander, Laura-Lee
1982 "Normal Aging" pp. 1-39 in Martha Logigian (ed.) Adult Rehabilitation: A Team Approach for Therapists Boston, MA: Little Brown & Co.

Madara, Edward
no   Developing Self-Help Groups - General Steps and Guidelines for Professionals
date   Denville, NJ: New Jersey Self-Help Clearinghouse

National Council on Disability
1986 Toward Independence: An Assessment of Federal Laws and Programs Affecting Persons with Disabilities - with Legislative Recommendations Washington DC: U.S. Government Printing Office

Roth, William
1981 The Handicapped Speak Jefferson, NC: McFarland

ORGANIZATIONS

(In the listings below, telephone numbers have symbols V for voice and TDD for tele-communication device for the deaf where organizations have published this information.)

Association for Advancement of Rehab Technology/RESNA
1101 Connecticut Avenue, NW, Suite 700
Washington DC 20036
(202) 857-1199

Multidisciplinary professional membership organization for people involved with improving technology for people with disabilities. Conducts a variety of projects, including research in the area of assistive technology and rehabilitation technology service delivery; technical assistance to statewide programs to develop technology. Membership. $95.00 includes "RESNA Newsletter."

Beach Center on Families and Disability
3111 Haworth Hall
University of Kansas
Lawrence KS 66045
(913) 864-7600

A federally funded center that conducts research and training in the factors that contribute to the successful functioning of families with members who have disabilities. Request a free publications catalog that describes monographs and tapes related to family coping, professional roles, and service delivery. Publishes newsletter, "Families and Disability," free.

Canadian Council on Social Concern Self-Help Unit
PO Box 3505, 55 Parkdale Avenue
Ottawa, Ontario K1Y 4G1 Canada
(613) 728-1865

Over 200 organizations throughout Canada participate in this self-help clearinghouse.

Canadian Rehabilitation Council for the Disabled (CRCD)
45 Sheppard Avenue East, Suite 801
Toronto, Ontario M2N 5W9 Canada
(416) 250-7490 (V/TDD)

A federation of regional and provincial groups that serve people with disabilities in Canada. Operates an information service and publishes a newsletter, "Access" and "Rehabilitation Digest" a quarterly journal with news about rehabilitation in Canada.

Combined Health Information Database (CHID)
Box NDIC (CHID)
Bethesda, MD 20892
(301) 468-2162

A federally operated database for service providers with bibliographic citations and abstracts from journals, reports, and education programs. Special files on arthritis, eye health, and diabetes.

Commission on Accreditation of Rehabilitation Facilities (CARF)
101 North Wilmot Road, Suite 500
Tucson, AZ 85711
(602) 748-1212 (V/TDD)

Conducts site evaluations and accredits organizations that provide rehabilitation.

Commission on Rehabilitation Counselor Certification
1835 Rohlwing Road, Suite E
Rolling Meadows, IL 60008
(708) 394-2104

Provides certification to rehabilitation counselors.

Independent Living Research Utilization (ILRU)
3400 Bissonnet, Suite 101
Houston, TX 77005
(713) 666-6244   (713) 666-0643 (TDD)

Develops and disseminates information; conducts training programs; sponsors conferences; and produces a wide variety of publications for people who administer independent living centers. Publishes a "Directory of Independent Living Programs," $8.50 (also available on audiocassette). Publishes a newsletter, "ILRU Insights," free.

Institute for Scientific Research (ISR)
33 Bedford Street, Suite 19A
Lexington, MA 02173
(617) 861-7900

Conducts research on the sociological aspects of disabilities and rehabilitation. Conducts evaluations of programs designed to train professionals and to rehabilitate individuals with disabilities.

National Association of Rehabilitation Facilities (NARF)
PO Box 17675
Washington DC 20041
(703) 648-9300

A national membership organization of individuals and institutions that provide rehabilitation services. Provides seminars, holds an annual meeting, and publishes a series of newsletters.

National Clearinghouse of Rehabilitation Training Materials (NCHRTM)
Oklahoma State University
816 West 6th Street
Stillwater, OK 74078
(405) 624-7650

Collects and disseminates publications and videos to train rehabilitation personnel. "NCHRTM Memo" describes the available materials.

National Council on Disability
800 Independence Avenue SW, Suite 814
Washington DC 20591
(202) 267-3846 (V)   (202) 267-3232 (TDD)

An independent federal agency mandated to study and make recommendations about public policy for people with disabilities. Holds regular meetings and hearings in various locations around the country. Publishes newsletter, "Focus," available in standard print, large print, or on audiocassette. Free

National Council on Independent Living (NCIL)
2539 Telegraph Avenue
Berkeley, CA 94704
(415) 849-1243

Advocates on behalf of people with disabilities and independent living centers that are controlled by people with disabilities. Provides information and referral, technical assistance, and a computer bulletin board. Membership, individuals, $35.00; organizations with voting rights, ranges from $125.00 to $600.00 depending on organization's budget; associate organization (no voting rights) $65.00. Membership includes quarterly "NCIL Newsletter," and bimonthly "President's Newsletter."

National Health Information Center
PO Box 1133
Washington DC 20013-1133
(800) 336-4797   In Maryland, (301) 565-4167

Maintains a database of health-related organizations and a library. Provides referrals related to health issues for both professionals and consumers. Publications enable individuals to locate information and resources in the federal government. Free publication list.

National Institute on Disability and Rehabilitation Research (NIDRR)
U.S. Department of Education
400 Maryland Avenue, SW
Washington DC 20202
(202) 732-1207   (202) 732-1198 (TDD)

A federal agency that supports research into various aspects of disability and rehabilitation, including demographic analyses, social science research, and the development of assistive devices. Grant programs are announced in the "Federal Register" or may be obtained directly from NIDRR.

National Organization on Disability (NOD)
910 16th Street, NW, Suite 600
Washington DC 20006
(800) 248-2253   (202) 293-5960 (V)   (202) 293-5968 (TDD)

An organization dedicated to achieving the full participation of people with disabilities in all aspects of community life. Works with a network of local agencies to achieve this goal. Provides technical assistance and maintains an informational database. Publishes newsletter, "Report."

National Rehabilitation Association (NRA)
633 South Washington
Alexandria, VA 22314-4193
(703) 836-0850

A professional membership organization for rehabilitation professionals and independent living center affiliates. Special opportunities for consumers and family members as well as students. Regular membership, $65.00, includes "Journal of Rehabilitation" and "NRA Newsletter;" student, consumer, family membership, $10.00

National Rehabilitation Information Center (NARIC)
8455 Colesville Road, Suite 935
Silver Spring, MD 20910-3319
(800) 346-2742   (301) 588-9284 (V/TDD)

A federally funded center that responds to telephone and mail inquiries about disabilities and support services. Maintains REHABDATA, a database with publications and research references. Publishes a newsletter, "NARIC Quarterly," free.

National Self-Help Clearinghouse
Graduate School and University Center/CUNY
33 West 42nd Street
New York, NY 10036
(212) 642-2944

A clearinghouse that makes referrals to self-help groups throughout the nation. Publishes newsletter, "The Self-Help Reporter."

New Jersey Self-Help Clearinghouse
St. Clare's Community Mental Health Center
Denville, NJ 07834
(201) 625-7101   (201) 625-9053 (TDD)   In NJ, (800) 367-6274

A clearinghouse that makes referrals to self-help groups throughout the nation. Publishes a variety of materials that are helpful to professionals and consumers who would like to start self-help groups, including "Ideas and Considerations for Starting a Self-Help Mutual Aid Group," "Suggestions on Locating a Meeting Place," and "Suggested Techniques for Recruiting Group Members."

Research and Training Center on Rural Rehabilitation
52 Corbin Hall
University of Montana
Missoula, MT 59812
(800) 723-0323   (406) 243-5467

A federally funded center that conducts research and training on issues that affect service delivery of rehabilitation in rural areas. Maintains a directory of rural disability services throughout the country. Publishes a quarterly newsletter, "RTC: Rural," free.

Research and Training Program on Independent Living (RTC/IL)
University of Kansas
4089 Dole
Lawrence, KS 66045
(913) 864-4095

A federally funded center that conducts research and training on the variables that affect independent living.

Resources for Rehabilitation
33 Bedford Street, Suite 19A
Lexington, MA 02173
(617) 862-6455

A private nonprofit organization that provides training and information to professionals who serve people with disabilities and to the public. Publications, training programs, program evaluations, and needs assessments. (See "PUBLICATIONS AND TAPES" section below.)

Society for Disability Studies (SDS)
14608 Melinda Avenue
Rockville, MD 20853
(301) 460-5963

Membership organization of practitioners, clinicians, and social scientists interested in the study of issues related to disability. Holds an annual meeting. Membership fee varies by income level. Discount on "Disability Studies Quarterly" (see "PUBLICATIONS AND TAPES" section below) as part of membership benefits.

TASH: The Association for Persons with Severe Handicaps
7010 Roosevelt Way, NE
Seattle, WA 98115
(206) 523-8446

A national advocacy organization that disseminates information to improve the education and increase the independence of individuals with severe disabilities. Holds an annual conference. Publishes a quarterly journal, "Journal of the Association for Persons with Severe Handicaps" and the "TASH Newsletter" (both included with membership). Regular membership, $72.00; parent/student/paraprofessional membership, $49.00.

United Way of America (UW)
701 North Fairfax Street
Alexandria, VA 22314-2045
(703) 836-7100

United Way/Centraide Canada
600-150 Kent
Ottawa, Ontario K1P 5P4 Canada
(613) 236-7041

An umbrella organization which links local human service organizations. National offices in the U.S. and Canada can direct you to the local UW which will provide referral to specific services in your community.

Vocational Rehabilitation Services
Veterans Benefits Administration
Department of Veterans Affairs (VA)
810 Vermont Avenue, NW
Washington DC 20420
(202) 233-6496

Provides education and rehabilitation assistance and independent living services to veterans with service related disabilities through offices located in every state as well as regional centers, medical centers, and insurance centers. Medical services are provided at VA Medical Centers, Outpatient Clinics, Domiciliaries, and Nursing Homes.

Well Spouse Foundation
PO Box 28876
San Diego, CA 92128

A network of support groups that provide emotional support to spouses and children of people who are chronically ill. Publishes a quarterly newsletter, "Well Spouse Foundation Newsletter," included in individual membership of $12.00; professional membership, $25.00.

World Institute on Disability (WID)
510 Sixteenth Street, Suite 100
Oakland, CA 94612
(415) 763-4100 (V/TDD)

WID is a public policy center founded and operated by individuals with disabilities. It conducts research, public education, and training and develops model programs related to disability. It deals with issues such as personal assistance, public transportation, employment, and access to health care. WID's Research and Training Center on Public Policy in Independent Living (PPIL) is a federally funded center that studies personal assistance services, federal independent living initiatives, and community integration issues.

Accent on Living
PO Box 700
Bloomington, IL 61702

A magazine with articles, product information, and tips on everyday living. Subscription, one year, $8.00; two years, $12.00; add $1.50 for Canada. Also publishes "Accent on Living Buyer's Guide," $10.00.

American Rehabilitation
Superintendent of Documents
U.S. Government Printing Office
Washington DC 20402

Published by the Rehabilitation Services Administration, this magazine covers a broad spectrum of issues related to rehabilitation, new publications, and news announcements. Published quarterly. $5.00 domestic, $6.25 foreign. Taped copies available from the National Library Service for the Blind and Physically Handicapped (See listing in Chapter 11, "Visual Impairment and Blindness").

Disability Studies Quarterly
Sociology Department
Brandeis University
Waltham, MA 02254

A quarterly journal with reports on recent research findings, upcoming meetings, grant solicitations. Book and audiovisual reviews. Individual subscription rate, $20.00

Federal Register
Superintendent of Documents
U.S. Government Printing Office
Washington DC 200402
(202) 783-3228

A federal publication printed every weekday with notices of all regulations and legal notices issued by federal agencies. Domestic subscriptions $340.00 annually for second class mailing of paper format; $195.00 annually for microfiche.

First Dibs
Box 1285
Tucson, AZ 85702-1285

A bimonthly newsletter with information about publications, products, conferences. $18.00

Foundations of the Vocational Rehabilitation Process
by Stanford E. Rubin and Richard T. Roessler
Pro-Ed
8700 Shoal Creek Boulevard
Austin, TX 78758-6897

A textbook with complete coverage of the development of vocational rehabilitation programs in the United States, legislative history, and procedures used by professionals to conduct client assessments and deliver services. $28.00

Independent Living
PO Box 202
Centerport, NY 11721

A magazine with articles, legislative news, and information about products that help people with disabilities. Free to service providers and consumers.

Journal of Disability Policy Studies
Department of Rehabilitation Education and Research
346 North West Avenue
Fayetteville, AR 72701
(501) 575-3656 (V/TDD)

A quarterly journal with articles related to legislative policy and regulatory matters as well as articles from a range of academic disciplines. Subscription, individuals, $24.50; institutions, $44.50

Journal of Rehabilitation
National Rehabilitation Association (NRA)
633 South Washington
Alexandria, VA 22314-4193
(703) 836-0850

A quarterly journal with articles related to the provision of rehabilitation services, psychological responses to disabilities, and book reviews. Subscription, U.S., $35.00; Canada, $40.00. Included in membership fee for National Rehabilitation Association (see "ORGANIZATIONS" section above).

Journal of Rehabilitation Research and Development (JRRD)
Office of Technology Transfer
VA Prosthetics R&D Center
103 South Gay Street
Baltimore, MD 21202

A quarterly publication of scientific and engineering articles related to spinal cord injury, prosthetics and orthotics, sensory aids, and gerontology. Includes abstracts of literature, book reviews, and calendar of events. For sale by U.S. Superintendent of Documents, Government Printing Office, Washington DC 20402

Mainstream
PO Box 370598
San Diego, CA 92137-0598

A magazine with articles, information about products, and a calendar of events. Subscription, one year, $16.98; two years, $32.00.

National Self-Help Network News
CEF Crisis/Helpline, Inc.
36 Brinkerhoff Street
Plattsburgh, NY 12901
(518) 561-2330

Provides information and resources to self-help groups and advocates. Free

Perspectives on Disability
Mark Nagler (ed.)
Health Markets Research
851 Moana Court
Palo Alto, CA 94306
(415) 948-1960

A collection of articles about attitudes, social interactions, the family, education, and medical and legal issues related to disability. Softcover, $60.00; hardcover $75.00

Report on Disability Programs
Business Publishers, Inc.
951 Pershing Drive
Silver Spring, MD 20910
(301) 587-6300

A biweekly newsletter reporting on government activities related to disabilities, disability programs around the nation, and a calendar of events. $213.50 for a year.

Unending Work and Care: Managing Chronic Illness at Home
by Juliet M. Corbin and Anselm Strauss
Jossey-Bass Inc.
350 Sansome Street
San Francisco, CA 94104

An analysis of the issues that affect the lives of individuals with chronic illness and their family members. Describes patients' physical and emotional needs; the role of health care personnel; and the means to manage chronic illness effectively. $35.95

Us and Them
Fanlight Productions
47 Halifax St.
Boston, MA 02130
(617) 524-0980

Videotape about relationships between people who have disabilities and those who do not. 32 minutes, black and white. Purchase, $275.00; rental for one day $50.00; for one week $100.00; plus $9.00 shipping charge

LAWS THAT AFFECT PEOPLE WITH DISABILITIES

(For laws specifically related to children and education, see Chapter 3, "Children and Youth")

Laws affecting people with disabilities cover a wide range of issues, including health care, financial benefits, housing, rehabilitation, civil rights, transportation, access to public buildings, and employment. For those who are not specialists in the law, it is sometimes difficult to keep abreast of the laws and their amendments. At the same time, people with disabilities may be able to continue living independently if they are aware of their rights and know how to locate the proper equipment and professional services. In many instances, government programs provide financial assistance for these needs.

In 1990, the *Americans with Disabilities Act* (ADA) was passed. Considered the most important piece of civil rights legislation in recent years, the ADA (P.L 101-336) will increase the steps employers must take to accommodate employees with disabilities and require that new buses and rail vehicles, facilities, and public accommodations be accessible. The major provisions of the ADA are as follows:

> • Prohibits discrimination against individuals with disabilities who are otherwise qualified for employment and requires that employers make "reasonable accommodations." "Reasonable accommodations" include making existing facilities accessible and job restructuring (e.g., including reassignment to a vacant position, modification of equipment, training, provision of interpreters and readers). Employers are protected from "undue hardship" in complying with this provision; the financial situation of the employer and the size and type of business are considered when determining whether an accommodation would constitute "undue hardship." Effective for employers with 25 or more employees two years after enactment of ADA and two years later for employers with 15 or more employees. (For a more detailed discussion of the employment aspects of the ADA, see Meeting the Needs of Employees with Disabilities, described in "PUBLICATIONS AND TAPES" section below).

> • Prohibits discrimination by public entities (i.e., local and state governments) and requires that individuals with disabilities be entitled to the same rights and benefits of public programs as other individuals.

• Requires that bus and railroad transportation systems address the needs of individuals with disabilities by purchasing adapted equipment, modifying facilities, and providing special transportation services that are comparable to regular transportation services.

• Requires that public accommodations, businesses, and services be accessible to individuals with disabilities. Public accommodations are broadly defined to include places such as hotels and motels, theatres, museums, schools, shopping centers and stores, banks, restaurants, and professional service providers' offices. After January 26, 1993, most new construction for public accommodations must be accessible to individuals with disabilities.

• Mandates that telephone companies provide relay services 24 hours a day, 7 days a week for individuals with hearing or speech impairments. Relay services enable individuals who have telecommunication devices for the deaf (TDD's) or another computer device that is capable of communicating across telephone lines to communicate with individuals who do not have such devices

Copies of the ADA are available from Senators and Representatives. Regulations for enforcing individual sections of the act are available from the federal agencies charged with promulgating them and in the "Federal Register" (see "PUBLICATIONS" section below). In addition, many private agencies that work with individuals with disabilities have copies of the ADA available for distribution to the public.

Agencies charged with formulating regulations and standards include the Architectural and Transportation Barriers Compliance Board, the Department of Transportation, the Equal Employment Opportunity Commission, the Federal Communications Commission, and the Attorney General. As this book went to press, some regulations had been published by the federal agencies charged with the enforcement of various sections of the law, but most had not yet been finalized.

Other major laws affecting people with disabilities include the **Rehabilitation Act of 1973** (P.L. 93-112) and its amendments, which are the centerpieces of federal law related to rehabilitation. States must submit a vocational rehabilitation plan to the Rehabilitation Services Administration indicating how the designated state agency will provide vocational training, counseling, and diagnostic and evaluation services required by the law. The "Client Assistance Program" authorizes states to inform clients and other persons with disabilities about all available benefits under the Act and to assist them in obtaining all remedies due under the law (P.L. 98-221). "Comprehensive Services for Independent Living" (P.L. 95-602) expanded rehabilitation services to severely disabled individuals, regardless of their vocational potential, making services available to many people who are no longer in the work force. The act broadly defines services as any "service that will the enhance the ability of a handicapped individual to live independently or function within his family and community..." These services may include counseling, job placement, housing, funds to make the home accessible, funds for prosthetic devices, attendant care, and recreational activities.

Section 503 of the Rehabilitation Act requires any contractor that receives more than $2,500 in contracts from the federal government to take affirmative action to employ individuals with disabilities. The Office of Federal Contract Compliance Programs within the Department of Labor is responsible for enforcing this provision (see "ORGANIZATIONS" section below). Section 504 prohibits any program that receives federal financial assistance from discriminating against individuals with disabilities who are otherwise eligible to benefit from their programs. Virtually all educational institutions are affected by this law, including private postsecondary institutions which receive federal financial assistance under a wide variety of programs. Programs must be physically accessible to individuals with disabilities, and construction begun after implementation of the regulations (June 3, 1977) must be designed so that it is in compliance with standard specifications for accessibility. Federal agencies must develop an affirmative action plan for hiring, placing, and promoting individuals with disabilities and for making their facilities accessible. The Civil Rights Division of the Department of Justice is responsible for enforcing this section.

Supplementary Security Income (SSI) is a federal minimum income maintenance program for elders and individuals who are blind or disabled and who meet a test of financial need. Monthly *Social Security Disability Insurance* (SSDI) benefits are available to individuals who are disabled and their dependents. To be eligible, individuals must have paid Social Security taxes for a specified number of years (dependent upon the applicant's age); must not be working; and must be declared medically disabled by the state disability determination service or through an appeals process. The disability must be expected to last at least 12 months or to result in death. Individuals who are blind and age 55 to 65 may receive monthly benefits if they are unable to carry out the work (or similar work) that they did before age 55 or becoming blind, whichever is later. Individuals who apply for disability insurance from the Social Security Administration must undergo an evaluation carried out by a state disability evaluation team, composed of physicians, psychologists, and other health care professionals. Social security disability benefits are not retroactive, so it is important to apply for them immediately after becoming disabled.

Individuals who have received SSDI for two consecutive years are eligible for *Medicare*, a federal health insurance program, which may cover some of the necessary out-patient therapy or supplies discussed in this book. However, Medicare does not cover eyeglasses, low vision aids, or hearing aids. *Medicaid* is a health insurance plan for individuals who are considered financially needy (i.e., recipients of financial benefits from governmental assistance programs such as Aid to Families with Dependent Children or Supplemental Security Income).

Medicaid is a joint federal/state program. While federal law requires that each state cover hospital services, skilled nursing facility services, physician and home health care services, and diagnostic and screening services, states have great discretion in other areas.

Payments for prosthetics and rehabilitation equipment vary greatly from state to state.

The medical and social service benefits available from organizations receiving federal assistance are guaranteed by federal laws and protected by the Office of Civil Rights of the Department of Health and Human Services (HHS). When an individual feels that his or her rights have been violated, a complaint should be filed with the regional office of HHS (see "ORGANIZATIONS" section below).

The *Technology-Related Assistance for Individuals with Disabilities Act* (P.L. 100-407) was passed in 1988. The Act mandates state-wide programs for technology related assistance to determine needs and resources; to provide technical assistance and information; and to develop demonstration and innovation projects, training programs, and public awareness programs. A copy of the law is available for $1.00 from The Superintendent of Documents, Government Printing Office, Washington DC 20402 (Stock # 869-006-00165-0).

Under amendments to the *Housing and Community Development Act of 1987* (P.L. 100-242), the Department of Housing and Urban Development (HUD) provides direct loans for the development of projects for elders and individuals with disabilities. These developments may consist of apartments or group homes for up to 15 residents. The *Fair Housing Amendments Act of 1988* (P.L. 100-430) requires that multifamily dwellings designed for first occupancy after March 13, 1991 be accessible to individuals with disabilities. In addition, HUD has established programs to house individuals with disabilities who are homeless.

The federal government allows special tax credits for people who are totally disabled and additional standard deductions for those who are legally blind. Legal blindness is defined as acuity of 20/200 or less in the better eye with the best possible correction or a field of 20 degrees or less diameter in the better eye. Tax deductions for business expenses include disability related expenditures, and deductions for medical expenses include special equipment such as wheelchairs, telecommunications devices for the deaf, and the like. Contact the Internal Revenue Service (see "ORGANIZATIONS" section below) to obtain publications that explain these benefits, including Publication 501, "Exemptions, Standard Deduction," and Filing Information, and Publication 524, "Credit for the Elderly or the Disabled."

All states and many local governments have adopted their own laws regarding accessibility. Information about these laws may be obtained from the state or local office serving people with disabilities. In many areas, special legal services for people with disabilities are available, often with fees on a sliding scale. Check with the local bar association or with a law school in your area. Some lawyers specialize in the legal needs of people with disabilities.

ORGANIZATIONS

(In the listings below, telephone numbers have symbols V for voice and TDD for tele-communication device for the deaf where organizations have published this information.)

Architectural and Transportation Barriers Compliance Board
1111 18th Street, NW, Suite 501
Washington DC 20036-3894
(800) 872-2253 (V/TDD)   (202) 653-7834 (V/TDD)

A federal agency charged with developing standards for accessibility in federal facilities, public accommodations, and transportation facilities as required by the Americans with Disabilities Act and other federal laws. Publishes the "Uniform Federal Accessibility Standards," which describes accessibility standards for buildings and dwelling units developed for four federal agencies. Provides technical assistance, sponsors research, and distributes publications. Publishes a free quarterly newsletter, "Access America." Publications available in standard print, large print, braille, audiocassette, and computer disk.

Clearinghouse on Disability Information
Office of Special Education and Rehabilitation Services (OSERS)
Room 3132, Switzer Building
Washington DC 20202-2524
(202) 732-1723

Responds to inquiries about federal legislation and programs for people with disabilities and makes referrals. Publishes newsletter, "OSERS News in Print," free.

Department of Housing and Urban Development (HUD)
Special Advisor for Disability Issues
Washington DC 20410-0001
(202) 426-6030 (V/TDD)

Operates programs to make housing accessible, including loans for developers of independent living and group homes and loan and mortgage insurance for rehabilitation of single or multifamily units. Free information kit.

Disability Rights Education and Defense Fund (DREDF)
2212 Sixth Street
Berkeley, CA 94710
(415) 644-2555   (415) 644-2626 (TDD)

Provides technical assistance, information, and referrals on laws and rights to callers; provides legal representation to people with disabilities in both individual and class action cases; trains law students, parents, and legislators.

Equal Employment Opportunity Commission (EEOC)
1801 L Street, NW, 10th floor
Washington DC 20507
(202) 663-4669 (V)   (202) 663-7026 (TDD)

Responsible for promulgating regulations for the employment section of the ADA. Copies of its regulations are available in standard print, large print, braille, computer disk, and audio-cassette.

Federal Communications Commission (FCC)
Washington DC 20554
(202) 632-7260

Responsible for developing regulations related to telephone relay services and other requirements of the ADA as it applies to telecommunications.

Internal Revenue Service (IRS)
(800) 829-3676

To receive Publication 501, "Exemptions, Standard Deduction," and Filing Information, and Publication 524, "Credit for the Elderly or the Disabled," call the number listed above.

National Council on Disability
800 Independence Avenue SW, Suite 814
Washington DC 20591
(202) 267-3846 (V)   (202) 267-3232 (TDD)

An independent federal agency mandated to study and make recommendations about public policy for people with disabilities. Holds regular meetings and hearings in various locations around the country. Publishes newsletter, "Focus," available in standard print, large print, or on audiocassette. Free

National Disability Action Center (NDAC)
2021 L Street, NW, Suite 800
Washington DC 20036
(202) 467-5730

An advocacy organization, NDAC drafts legislation to increase the accessibility for individuals with disabilities and represents people with disabilities who have been the target of discrimination.

Office of Civil Rights
Department of Education
300 C Street, SW
Washington DC 20202
(202) 732-1213

Responsible for enforcing laws and regulations designed to protect the rights of individuals in educational institutions that receive federal financial assistance. Individuals who feel their rights have been violated may file a complaint with one of the ten regional offices located throughout the country.

Office of Civil Rights
Department of Health and Human Services
330 Independence Avenue, SW (Cohen Building)
Washington DC 20201
(202) 619-0585

Responsible for enforcing laws and regulations designed to protect the rights of individuals who are seeking medical and social services in institutions that receive federal financial assistance. Individuals who feel their rights have been violated may file a complaint with one of the ten regional offices located throughout the country.

Office of Federal Contract Compliance Programs
Department of Labor
Employment Standards Administration
200 Constitution Avenue, NW, Room C-3325
Washington DC 20210
(202) 523-9476

Reviews contractors' affirmative action plans, provides technical assistance to contractors, investigates complaints and resolves issues between contractors and employees. Ten regional offices throughout the country serve as liaisons with the national office and with district offices under their jurisdiction.

Office of Transportation Regulatory Affairs
Department of Transportation
400 Seventh Street, SW
Washington DC 20590
(202) 366-9306 (V)   (202) 755-7687 (TDD)

Responsible for promulgating regulations for transportation of individuals with disabilities required by the Rehabilitation Act and the Americans with Disabilities Act. Regulations available in standard print or on audiocassette.

<u>Office on the Americans with Disabilities Act</u>
Civil Rights Division
Department of Justice
PO Box 66118
Washington DC 20035-6118
(202) 514-0301 (V)   (202) 514-0381 (TDD)   (202) 514-0383 (TDD)

Responsible for enforcing the Americans with Disabilities Act. Copies of its regulations are available in standard print, large print, braille, computer disk, audiocassette, and on an electronic bulletin board [(202) 514-6193].

<u>Social Security Administration</u>
Department of Health and Human Services
Baltimore, MD 21235
(800) 234-5772

To apply for social security benefits based on disability, phone the number above to set up an appointment with a social security representative, or visit the social security office nearest to your home. The Office of Disability within the Social Security Administration publishes "Social Security Regulations: Rules for Determining Disability and Blindness," free.

<u>Dis/ability Law Briefs</u>
American Bar Association Commission on the Mentally Disabled
1800 M Street, NW, Suite 200
Washington DC 20036

A quarterly newsletter for professionals and consumers. Reports on programs, publications, and news affecting people with disabilities. Free

<u>Disability Rights Guide</u>
by Charles D. Goldman
Media Publishing/MPM, Inc
2440 O Street, Suite 202
Lincoln, NE 68510-1125

A summary and simplification of laws related to disability. Includes chapters on housing, accessibility, and transportation. $14.95 plus $2.00 shipping

<u>Federal Register</u>
Superintendent of Documents
U.S. Government Printing Office
Washington DC 200402
(202) 783-3228

A federal publication printed every weekday with notices of all regulations and legal notices issued by federal agencies. Domestic subscriptions $340.00 annually for second class mailing of paper format; $195.00 annually for microfiche.

<u>Meeting the Needs of Employees with Disabilities</u>
Resources for Rehabilitation
33 Bedford Street, Suite 19A
Lexington, MA 02173
(617) 862-6455

Provides information to help people with disabilities retain or obtain employment. Information on government programs and laws, supported employment, training programs, environmental adaptations, and the transition from school to work are included. Chapters on mobility, vision, and hearing and speech impairments include information on organizations, products, and services that enable employers to accommodate the needs of employees with disabilities. $42.95 plus $5.00 shipping and handling (See order form opposite inside back cover.)

Mental and Physical Disability Law Reporter
American Bar Association Commission on the Mentally Disabled
1800 M Street, NW, Suite 200
Washington DC 20036

A bimonthly journal with court decisions, legislative and regulatory news, and articles on treatment, accessibility, employment, education, federal programs, etc. Individual subscription, $140.00; organizational subscription, $195.00

Pocket Guide to Federal Help for Individuals with Disabilities
Consumer Information Center
Pueblo, CO 81002

A summary of benefits and services available from the federal government. Request publication 119V, $1.00

SSI & Social Security Disability: Securing and Protecting Your Benefits
Protection & Advocacy, Inc.
175 West Jackson, # A-2103
Chicago, IL 60604
(312) 341-0022 (V/TDD)

A booklet describing eligibility for benefits, the application and appeals process, work incentive programs, and finding an attorney or advocate. Free

Summary of Existing Legislation Affecting Persons with Disabilities
Office of Special Education and Rehabilitation Services (OSERS)
Clearinghouse on Disability Information
Room 3132, Switzer Building
Washington DC 20202-2524

Published in 1988, this book includes sections on income maintenance programs, health, housing, vocational rehabilitation, and transportation. Free

Toward Independence
National Council on Disability
800 Independence Avenue, SW, Suite 814
Washington DC 20591
(202) 267-3846 (V)   (202) 267-3232 (TDD)

A 1986 report to the U.S. Congress on the federal laws and programs serving people with disabilities and recommendations for legislation. Free

CHILDREN AND YOUTH

When parents learn that their child has a disability or chronic condition, they are often overwhelmed by their own emotional responses as well as the pressures of providing the child with the best possible medical and rehabilitation services. At a time when they often feel guilty, frightened about their child's future, and depressed, they must learn about a new system of services and how to integrate these services into their family life.

Parents are rarely prepared for this situation, unless by chance they have friends or family members who have dealt with a similar condition in their own family. How families cope with a child with a disability or chronic condition is influenced by a variety of factors, including educational level of parents, financial status, personality characteristics of family members, and the availability of services to help the child. Although some families may break up as a result of the stress caused by having a child with a disability or chronic condition, others become closer (Shapiro: 1983).

Because parents experience such intense emotional reactions to a child's disability or illness, counseling to help them cope with their own emotions will contribute to their ability to help the child. Such counseling may be available from medical professionals, social workers or psychologists, rehabilitation counselors, and other parents in similar situations. Talking with other parents either in private or at a parent support group helps parents to learn that their emotional responses are normal. Parent groups also serve as a mechanism to channel energy into productive ways of helping their child. Support groups, which in many cases are focused on a specific disability, help parents to learn about the services available for their child and how to effectively cope with the various professionals that they inevitably will deal with. In addition to providing information and referrals, parent groups may also have a system of providing respite care.

Teplin (1988) recommends that professionals discuss the parents' questions and concerns; recognize that early intervention and parent education are important for normal development; and recognize that the physician must take the initiative in making referrals to supportive agencies and resources. Failure to make referrals may cause the family to "flounder needlessly, while the infant misses valuable opportunities for cognitive, motor, and emotional development" (Teplin: 1988, 302). Teplin's ten roles for physicians to promote optimal development of children and infants who are blind may be used as guidelines by health care or rehabilitation professionals serving children with any disability or chronic condition.

Although numerous professionals may be involved in helping children with disabilities and chronic conditions, ultimately it is the parents' responsibility to ensure that their child receives optimal medical care, rehabilitation, and education. Gliedman and Roth make several suggestions to help parents achieve this goal, including:

  • Monitor your child's progress closely and keep copies of your child's records.

  • Keep records of visits with professionals, including dates, who was present, and what was said.

  • If you do not understand any terms that are used, ask for a translation into "lay" language.

  • Learn as much as you can about your child's condition.

  • Stay in touch with your child's teacher.

  • Listen to your child when he or she expresses individual needs (1980: pp. 184-185)

Stress factors which affect the families of children with a disability or chronic condition include financial problems, often caused by limitations of health insurance coverage; lack of information about medical and community services available; and the need to restructure the family itself. It is wise to schedule visits to physicians and other service providers' offices so that parents can share the responsibility for the child's care.

When other children are in the family, the situation is compounded by the need to preserve a sense of normalcy and at the same time help the child who has a disability or chronic condition. Siblings may be jealous of the attention which is paid to the child with a disability. They may feel embarrassed to have a sibling whose physical appearance or behavior is abnormal, and they may fear rejection by their peers. Siblings need information about the condition or disability which affects their sister or brother in order to be comfortable.

As the child develops and enters different environments, it is important for his or her peers to be educated about the disability or condition. Children must learn that individuals who are different should not be viewed negatively. Children who do not have disabilities should be encouraged to ask adults questions about disabilities. They should be told that teasing will hurt the other child's feelings. Disability awareness programs in schools, religious organizations, and youth groups offer an opportunity to educate children about a specific disability or a range of conditions. The "Kids on the Block" puppets (see "ORGANIZATIONS" section below) and programs which enable children to simulate an experience with a disability encourage understanding and acceptance.

Children with a disability or chronic condition often benefit from participation in programs which match them with role models. Partners for Disabled Youth (see "ORGANIZATIONS" section below) matches adults and youngsters with disabilities in a big brother/big sister relationship. The adults share their life experiences and provide a sounding board for questions about school, recreation, employment, social life, and many other issues. Working with these youngsters gives the adults an opportunity to share their life experience, provide inspiration, and to give something back to the community.

Children and youth with disabilities and chronic conditions use a wide variety of adaptive aids at home, in the classroom, and in recreation. Many specialized aids have been developed to make independent learning and living safe and comfortable. Often family members, teachers, or other professionals create assistive devices to meet a particular need.

LAWS AND EDUCATION

The enactment of the *Education of the Handicapped Act* (P.L. 94-142) in 1975 broke ground for the expansion of educational services for children with disabilities and established legal rights for these children to obtain an appropriate education from the public school system. The law requires that states provide all children with disabilities an appropriate public education in the least restrictive setting. Special education services provided in public school classrooms, at home, and in hospitals and institutions are included. Related services that states must provide include transportation; physical, occupational, audiological, and speech therapy; and psychological services (U.S. Department of Education: 1988). In addition, the U.S. Department of Education is mandated to provide funding for a variety of programs that train special educators and other professional personnel to serve children with special needs.

In order for states to receive federal funding for programs for children with disabilities, the state department of education must establish a plan and procedures for providing these services and require that local educational agencies maintain individualized education plans (IEP's) for each child served. Federal funds are allocated to states based on the number of children with disabilities served. In the 1986-87 school year, 4.4 million children and youths (ages 3 to 21) received services mandated by this law and by the Education Consolidation and Improvement Act - State Operated Programs.

In addition, the federal law has mandated that regional resource centers be established to provide technical assistance to professional educators who provide services for children and youth with disabilities. These centers may be operated by a college or university, state or local education agency, or private nonprofit organization that has received a federal grant for this purpose. The state educational agency is required to publish a listing of the resource centers in the state.

The *Education of the Handicapped Act Amendments of 1983* (P.L. 98-199) expanded the incentives to local and state governments to provide equal educational opportunities in preschool, early intervention, and transition programs. The *Education of the Handicapped Act Amendments of 1986* (P.L. 99-457) lowered the eligibility for special education services to age three and established the Handicapped Infant and Toddler Programs (birth to age three). These programs provide early intervention services to infants and toddlers who have been diagnosed with physical or mental conditions for which there is a high probability of developmental delay (Center for Special Education Technology: 1991). States are required to develop a comprehensive, statewide, interagency service delivery system by their fifth year of participation in the program (National Information Center for Children and Youth with Disabilities: 1991).

In 1990, the name of the Education of the Handicapped Act was changed to the *Individuals with Disabilities Education Act*, referred to as IDEA (P.L. 101-476). IDEA expanded education programs to include services to children with serious emotional problems, attention deficits, autism, and traumatic brain injury.

Under the provisions of the various Acts cited above, the special education teacher, health care providers, and the parents work together to develop an Individualized Education Plan (IEP), which specifies educational goals, courses of instruction, special equipment, and other services to be provided. The IEP is based on the results of an individualized evaluation and assessment of the child. Schools are required to notify parents in writing any time a decision is made related to the identification of the child's disability, educational needs, development of the IEP, or placement in a special or regular program. Parents have the right to appeal if they disagree with the school's decision and may arrange for an independent evaluation of their child.

Adolescents with disabilities have special needs as they consider career goals and higher education. Vocational education offers students a combination of classroom instruction and practical job experience to develop the occupational skills needed in the labor market. Vocational education is available in high schools, community colleges, and technical institutes. The *Carl D. Perkins Vocational and Applied Technology Education Act* (P.L. 101-392) provides increased resources to achieve the academic and occupational skills necessary for employment in high technology. Individuals with disabilities are included in this mandate.

Section 504 of the Rehabilitation Act of 1973 prohibits any institution that receives federal funds from discriminating against people with disabilities. Since virtually all postsecondary institutions receive federal funds, they are required to comply with the regulations developed for the enforcement of Section 504 (See Chapter 2, "Laws that Affect People with Disabilities"). Students who qualify for admission into postsecondary education programs must be provided with the services that they need to complete their education (Bowe: 1987). Most universities, colleges and community colleges have established special offices to serve students with disabilities. Sources of financial assistance for postsecondary students with disabilities are listed below under "FINANCIAL AID FOR POSTSECONDARY EDUCATION."

34

References

Bowe, Frank G.
1987 "Section 504: 10 Years Later" American Rehabilitation (April/May/June):2-3;23-24

Center for Special Education Technology
1991 "Update: 1990 Demographic Data" The Marketplace: Report on Technology in Special Education 4:1

Gliedman, John and William Roth
1980 The Unexpected Minority: Handicapped Children in America New York, NY: Harcourt Brace Jovanovich

National Information Center for Children and Youth with Disabilities
1991 "The Education of Children and Youth with Special Needs: What Do the Laws Say?" NICHCY News Digest I:1

Shapiro, Johanna
1983 "Family Reactions and Coping Strategies in Response to the Physically Ill or Handicapped Child: A Review" Social Science and Medicine 17:14:913-931

Teplin, Stuart W.
1988 "Development of the Blind Infant and Child with Retinopathy of Prematurity: The Physician's Role in Intervention," pp. 301-323 in John T. Flynn and Dale L. Phelps (eds.) Retinopathy of Prematurity: Problem and Challenge New York, NY: Alan R. Liss, Inc.

U.S. Department of Education
1988 Summary of Existing Legislation Affection Persons with Disabilities Washington DC: Office of Special Education and Rehabilitative Services, Clearinghouse on the Handicapped, Publication No. E-88-22014

(In the listings below, telephone numbers have symbols V for voice and TDD for tele-communication device for the deaf where organizations have published this information.)

Administration on Developmental Disabilities (ADD)
U.S. Department of Health and Human Services
200 Independence Avenue, S.W.
Washington DC 20201
(202)245-2890

Works with state governments, local communities, and the private sector to promote self-sufficiency and protect the rights of individuals with developmental disabilities.

American Vocational Association
1410 King Street
Alexandria, VA 22314
(800) 826-9972   (703) 683-3111

Professional association for individuals who work in the field of vocational education. Many special divisions including a Special Needs Division and Technology Education Division. Publishes "Vocational Education Journal," included in membership fee of $40.00. Nonmembers, $20.00

Association for the Care of Children's Health
3615 Wisconsin Avenue, NW
Washington, DC 20016
(202) 244-1801

Multidisciplinary association of professionals and parents. Distributes "Books for Children and Teenagers About Hospitalization, Illness, and Disabling Conditions," by Lisa Redburn, an annotated bibliography. Members, $6.00; nonmembers, $9.00.

Association on Handicapped Student Service Programs in Postsecondary Education (AHSSPPE)
PO Box 21192
Columbus, OH 43221
(614) 488-4972 (V/TDD)

Promotes the full participation of individuals with disabilities in postsecondary education. Publishes the "Journal of Postsecondary Education and Disability," "ALERT Newsletter," proceedings of annual conferences, and other reference publications. Special interest groups focus on specific disabilities, technology, Canadian programs, and other topics. Regular membership, $75.00; other categories include affiliate, institutional, and student memberships.

Barrier-Free Design Centre
2075 Bayview Avenue
Toronto, Ontario M4N 3M5 Canada
(416) 480-6009

Provides education and technical consultation in barrier-free design and construction. Publishes professional guides and "The Accessible Home: Renovating for Your Disabled Child," $12.00 plus $3.00 shipping and handling (Canadian funds).

Beach Center on Families and Disability
Bureau of Child Research
University of Kansas
3111 Haworth Hall
Lawrence, KS 66045
(913) 864-7600

A federally funded center that conducts research and training about the functioning of families with members who have disabilities. Catalog describes monographs and tapes related to family coping, professional roles, and service delivery. Newsletter, "Families and Disability," free.

Clearinghouse on Disability Information
Office of Special Education and Rehabilitative Services (OSERS)
330 C Street, SW, Room 3132, Switzer Building
Washington, DC 20202-2524
(202) 732-1723

Federal information clearinghouse on disabilities. Quarterly newsletter, "OSERS News in Print," free.

Council for Exceptional Children (CEC)
1920 Association Drive
Reston, VA 22091
(703) 620-3660

A professional membership organization that works to improve the quality of education for children who are gifted or have disabilities. Holds annual conference. Regular membership, $55.00. Publishes abstracts of on-going research projects currently funded by the Division of Innovation and Development, Office of Special Education Programs, U.S. Department of Education. Manages ERIC Clearinghouse on Handicapped and Gifted, which answers telephone inquiries and provides handout materials. Publishes "Teaching Exceptional Children," a quarterly journal for special educators; U.S., $20.00; Canada, $23.00; and newsletter, "Exceptional Children," published bimonthly, $25.00. Also publishes "Journal of Special Education," available from Pro-Ed, 8700 Shoal Creek Boulevard, Austin, TX 78758-6897, (512) 451-8542. Individual subscription, $35.00; business subscription, $70.00.

National Association of State Directors of Special Education (NASDSE)
2021 K Street, NW, Suite 315
Washington, DC 20036-1003
(202) 296-1800

A coalition of state directors of special education. Published the entire text of the Individuals with Disabilities Education Act, including the 1990 amendments. $15.00

National Center for Research in Vocational Education
1995 University Avenue, Suite 375
Berkeley, CA 94704-1058
(800) 762-4093   (415) 642-4004

Conducts applied research and development in vocational education. Services include leadership development, in-service education, technical assistance for special populations, and publications.

National Center for Youth with Disabilities
Box 721 UMHC
Harvard Street at East River Road
Minneapolis, MN 55455
(800) 333-6293   (612) 626-2825

Provides information and technical assistance on the needs of adolescents and young adults with chronic illnesses and disabilities. National resource library available through computer database. "CYDLINE Reviews" are a series of annotated bibliographies on topics related to youth with disabilities; prices vary with content. Free quarterly newsletter, "Connections."

National Clearinghouse on Postsecondary Education for Individuals with Disabilities
HEATH Resource Center
One Dupont Circle, NW, Suite 800
Washington, DC 20036-1193
(800) 544-3284 (V/TDD)   In Washington DC area, (202) 939-9320

Provides information about the needs of youth in transition from high school to postsecondary education. Newsletter, "Information from HEATH," free. Fact sheets include "Career Planning and Placement Strategies for Postsecondary Students with Disabilities," "How to Choose a College: Guide for the Student with a Disability" and "Vocational Rehabilitation Services: A Postsecondary Student Consumer's Guide." Free publications list.

National Clearinghouse on Women and Girls with Disabilities
Educational Equity Concepts
114 East 32nd Street
New York, NY 10016
(212) 725-1803

Provides information, resources, and referrals. Publishes "Bridging the Gap: A National Directory of Services for Women and Girls with Disabilities," which lists organizations that serve girls and women with disabilities and resource information. Individuals, $15.00; organizations, $25.00.

National Committee for Citizens in Education
10840 Little Patuxent Parkway, Suite 301
Columbia, MD 21044
(800) 638-9675   (301) 997-9300

Provides information and technical assistance to parents and schools. Bimonthly newsletter "Network for Public Schools," reports on advocacy efforts, including advocacy for children with disabilities. "NCCE Catalog" accompanies newsletter. $12.00

National Information Center For Children and Youth with Disabilities (NICHCY)
PO Box 1492
Washington, DC 20013
(800) 999-5599   In Washington DC area, (703) 893-6061   (703) 893-8614 (TDD)

Clearinghouse which provides free information and referral, technical assistance, and publications to parents, educators, caregivers, and advocates. Newsletter, "News Digest," free.

National Library Service for the Blind and Physically Handicapped
1291 Taylor Street, NW
Washington, DC 20542
(800) 424-8567 or 8572

Provides free talking book equipment on loan and recorded and braille books for preschoolers, children, and adults with physical disabilities or visual impairment and blindness through a regional network of cooperating libraries. "Children and Teens" describes the services for young people with temporary or permanent disabilities. Three free bibliographies are "Parents' Guide to the Development of Preschool Handicapped Children: Resources and Services," "Selected Readings for Parents of Preschool Handicapped Children," and "From School to Working Life: Resources and Services."

National Maternal and Child Health Clearinghouse
38 and R Streets, NW
Washington, DC 20057
(800) 346-2742

Provides information on genetic disorders, genetic counseling, disabling conditions, child health and development, and other issues of maternal and child health. Publishes directories, bibliographies, and newsletters.

PACER Center (Parent Advocacy Coalition for Educational Rights)
4826 Chicago Avenue South
Minneapolis, MN 55417-1055
(612) 827-2966 (V/TDD)

A coalition of Minnesota disability organizations which provides parent training, programs for students and schools, technical assistance, and publications. Many publications are free to Minnesota residents; nominal fee for non-residents. Newsletter, "PACESETTER," free. Free catalogue of publications.

Partners for Disabled Youth
Massachusetts Office on Disability
One Ashburton Place
Boston, MA 02108
(617) 727-7440   In MA, (800) 322-2020

Matches adults and children with disabilities. Adult partners act as role models and mentors.

Sibling Information Network
University Affiliated Program
University of Connecticut
991 Main Street, Suite 3A
East Hartford, CT 06108
(203) 282-7050

Clearinghouse for information, literature, and research about siblings and other issues of families of individuals with disabilities. Quarterly "Sibling Information Network Newsletter," includes SIBPAGE, an insert written by and for siblings, ages 5 to 15. Free

TASH: The Association for Persons with Severe Handicaps
7010 Roosevelt Way, NE
Seattle, WA 98115
(206) 523-8446

Works to improve the education and increase the independence of individuals with severe disabilities. Holds annual conference. Quarterly "Journal of the Association for Persons with Severe Handicaps" and "TASH Newsletter" (both included with membership). Regular membership, $72.00; student/paraprofessional/parent membership, $49.00.

Technical Assistance for Special Populations Program (TASPP)
1310 South Sixth Street
Champaign, IL 61820
(217) 333-0807

Provides resource and referral services to professionals working with individuals with special needs at secondary and postsecondary levels. Publishes free "BRIEFS," which highlight critical vocational education issues; newsletter, "TASPP Bulletin;" and offers free information searches on a computerized database.

Technical Assistance to Parent Programs (TAPP) Network
Federation for Children with Special Needs
95 Berkeley Street, Suite 104
Boston, MA 02116
(617) 482-2915 (V/TDD)   In MA, (800) 331-0688

Provides technical assistance in health issues through parent training and information activities. Newsletter, "Coalition Quarterly," free.

<u>After the Tears: Parents Talk About Raising a Child with a Disability</u>
by Robin Simons
TASH (The Association for Persons with Severe Handicaps)
7010 Roosevelt Way, NE
Seattle, WA 98115
(206) 523-8446

Describes how parents face the challenges of raising a child with a disability, from initial shock and grief to recovery. $8.00

<u>Apple Computer Resources in Special Education and Rehabilitation</u>
c/o DLM Teaching Resources
One DLM Park
Allen, TX 75002
(800) 527-4747

Describes more than 1,000 hardware and software products, publications, and organizations for children and adults with disabilities. $19.95 plus $2.00 shipping and handling

<u>Directory of College Facilities and Services for People with Disabilities</u>
James L. Thomas and Carol H. Thomas (eds.)
Oryx Press, Phoenix, AZ
(800) 279-6799

Provides information on the special services and facilities available for students with disabilities at colleges and universities in the United States and Canada. $115.00

<u>Disability and the Family: A Guide to Decisions for Adulthood</u>
by H. Rutherford Turnbull III, Ann P. Turnbull, G.J. Bronicki, Jean Ann Summers, and Constance Roeder-Gordon
Brookes Publishing Company
PO Box 10624
Baltimore, MD 21285-9945
(800) 638-3775

Provides guidance in planning for the future of an individual with a disability. Legal, financial, recreational, and vocational options are discussed. $29.00

<u>Early Childhood Reporter</u>
LRP Publications
747 Dresher Road
PO Box 980
Horsham, PA 19044-0980
(800) 341-7874

Monthly reports with information on federal, state, and local legislation affecting the implementation of early intervention and preschool programs for children with disabilities. $125.00.

<u>Exceptional Parent</u>
Psy-Ed Corporation
PO Box 3000, Department EP
Denville, NJ 07834
(800) 247-8080

This magazine emphasizes problem solving and provides practical information about dealing with a child with a disability. 8 issues per year, $18.00.

<u>Kaleidoscope</u>
University-Affiliated Program on Developmental Disabilities
University of Connecticut
991 Main Street
Hartford, CT 06108
(203) 282-7050

Written for families of individuals with developmental disabilities, this quarterly newsletter includes information about literature, films, and research. Individuals, $5.00; organizations, $15.00.

<u>The Kids on the Block</u>
9385-C Gerwig Lane
Columbia, MD 21046
(800) 368-5437   (301) 290-9095

Puppets are used to help students understand disabilities and chronic conditions. Various programs available. Also publishes "The Kids on the Block" series of books, written for children in grades two to five, which feature children with chronic conditions or disabilities such as diabetes, epilepsy, and visual impairment. Question and answer sections about the characters' disabilities in each book. $12.95

<u>Making the Transition: A Guide for Helping Students with Special Needs</u>
American Vocational Association
Department 1090
1410 King Street
Alexandria, VA 22314
(800) 826-9972   (703) 683-3111

Discusses techniques which help students with disabilities make the transition from school to work. Members, $10.95; nonmembers, $12.95.

<u>1990 Guide to Department of Education Programs</u>
Superintendent of Documents
U.S. Government Printing Office
Washington, DC 20402

Lists all Department of Education programs including special education and rehabilitative services. Free

<u>A Parents' Guide to Accessing Parent Groups, Community Services, and to Keeping Records</u>
National Information Center for Children and Youth with Disabilities
PO Box 1492
Washington, DC 20013
(800) 999-5599   In Washington DC area, (703) 893-6061   (703) 893-8614 (TDD)

Provides guidelines for locating and/or organizing parent groups; describes community services and how to use them; includes a special section for rural families; and makes recommendations for organizing medical, school, and community services records. Free

<u>A Reader's Guide for Parents of Children with Mental, Physical, or Emotional Disabilities</u>
Woodbine House
5615 Fishers Lane
Rockville, MD 20852
(800) 843-7323

An annotated bibliography which provides information about disabilities, advocacy, books for children about disabilities, and reference sources for families. $14.95

<u>Respite Care: A Guide for Parents</u> $4.00
<u>Respite Care is for Families: A Guide to Program Development</u> $4.00
CSR, Incorporated
Respite
1400 Eye Street, NW, Suite 600
Washington, DC 20005
(202) 842-7600

44

Resource guides for families and service providers to help them locate or develop respite care programs.

Someday's Child
What About Me
Educational Productions Inc.
7412 SW Beaverton Hillsdale Highway, Suite 210
Portland, OR 97225
(800) 950-4949   (503) 292-9234

Videotapes for children and families with special needs. "Someday's Child" gives three families' perspectives on raising children with disabilities. "What About Me?" presents interviews with siblings of children with disabilities and shows a sibling support group meeting at which brothers and sisters express their feelings about family life. Facilitator and viewer discussion guides accompany videos. Each tape: 2 week preview, $35.00; $250.00 to purchase.

Steps to Independence: A Skills Training Guide for Parents and Teachers of Children with Special Needs
by Bruce L. Baker and Alan J. Brightman
Brookes Publishing Company
PO Box 10624
Baltimore, MD 21285-9945
(800) 638-3775

A resource guide for teaching independent living. Includes sample activities, self-help sources, and case examples. $24.00

Vocational Education for the Disadvantaged & Handicapped: A Guide to Program Administration
American Vocational Association
1410 King Street, Department 1090
Alexandria, VA 22314
(800) 826-9972   (703) 683-3111

Makes recommendations for implementation of the Perkins Vocational and Applied Technology Education Act. Members, $10.95; nonmembers, $12.95.

College: The Basics
National Center for Postsecondary Governance and Finance
University of Maryland Foundation
4114 CSS Building
College Park, MD 20742
(301) 405-5582

A set of audio tapes that discusses financial aid in general, for students with disabilities, and other issues. Printed contact information included. $14.95

The Federal Educational and Scholarship Funding Guide
Grayco Publishing
PO Box 1291
West Warwick, RI 02893

Lists more than 125 organizations that make grants in all aspects of education. $39.95

Federal Student Aid
Federal Student Aid Center
PO Box 84
Washington, DC 20044

This cassette describes financial aid available to students with vision loss; includes federal grant, loan, and work-study programs; scholarships; and discusses the rights of students with disabilities. Free

Financial Aid for Students with Disabilities
HEATH Resource Center
One Dupont Circle
Washington, DC 20036-1193
(800) 544-3284

Covers grants, loans, and work-study programs; vocational rehabilitation services; and organizations that provide scholarships. Free

Financial Aid for the Disabled and Their Families
by Gail Ann Schlachter and R. David Weber
Reference Service Press
1100 Industrial Road, Suite 9
San Carlos, CA 94070

Lists scholarships, loans, grants, awards, and internships. $35.00 plus $3.00 shipping

MAKING EVERYDAY LIVING EASIER

Individuals with disabilities and chronic conditions use a wide variety of adaptive aids which enable them to continue with their everyday activities. Many ingenious aids have been developed to make independent living safe and comfortable. Often individuals create assistive devices to meet their own needs. Hand-in-hand with a growing sense of independence among individuals with disabilities is the desire to participate in travel and recreational activities.

This chapter is divided into two sections. "Environmental Adaptations and Assistive Devices" describes organizations and publications with information about adaptations for the home and aids for use in everyday living. "Travel and Recreation" describes general resources; refer to earlier chapters for information on a specific disability (e.g.,travelers with diabetes).

ENVIRONMENTAL ADAPTATIONS AND ASSISTIVE DEVICES

Housing adaptations range from the installation of a ramp or simple tactile markings in elevators to major renovations, which include elevators and special appliances. Many architects now specialize in designing buildings and dwelling units that meet the needs of people with disabilities.

Although some of the publications described below mention a specific disability or age, they include suggestions that are applicable for individuals of all ages and with a variety of conditions. Suppliers of personal and home health care aids, recreational products, and mobility aids for more than one type of condition or disability are listed. For suppliers of adaptive aids for a specific disability or condition, refer to the chapter that deals with that disability or condition (e.g., vision loss, hearing loss, etc.). Many hospital pharmacies as well as large department and discount stores now sell home health products such as wheelchairs, bathroom safety devices, canes, and walkers. Some of this equipment may also be available on a rental or loan basis from community health agencies.

(In the listings below, telephone numbers have symbols V for voice and TDD for telecommunication device for the deaf where organizations have published this information.)

ABLEDATA
Adaptive Equipment Center
Newington Children's Hospital
181 East Cedar Street
Newington, CT 06111
(800) 344-5405 (V/TDD)   In CT, (203) 667-5405 (V/TDD)

Disability-related products for personal care, recreation, and transportation are listed in a database. First eight pages of database searches, free; a fee is charged for longer searches.

Accent on Living
PO Box 700
Bloomington, IL 61702
(309) 378-2961

A database of assistive devices and how-to information. Publishes "Accent on Living," a quarterly magazine, $8.00 per year, and "Accent on Living Buyers' Guide," $10.95

American Institute on Architects (AIA)
1735 New York Avenue, NW
Washington, DC 20006
(202) 626-7300

Professional membership organization. Publishes two bibliographies related to disabilities: one of books in AIA Reference Library (number B 100) and one of periodical article citations (number P 131) on barrier-free design. Free for members; nonmembers, $15.00 per bibliography. "Americans with Disabilities Act Information Kit" describes the ADA's effect on the field of architecture; members, $9.95; nonmembers, $16.95.

Architectural and Transportation Barriers Compliance Board
1111 18th Street, NW, Suite 501
Washington DC 20036-3894
(800) 872-2253 (V/TDD)   (202) 653-7834 (V/TDD)

A federal agency charged with developing standards for accessibility. Provides technical assistance, sponsors research, and distributes publications. Publishes a free quarterly newsletter, "Access America." Publications available in standard print, large print, braille, audio-tape, and computer disk.

Barrier-Free Design Centre
2075 Bayview Avenue
Toronto, Ontario M4N 3M5 Canada
(416) 480-6009

Provides education, information, and technical consultation in barrier-free design and construction for Canadians with disabilities. Publishes professional guides for barrier-free design and "The Accessible Home: Renovating for Your Disabled Child," $12.00 plus $3.00 shipping and handling (Canadian funds).

Center for Accessible Housing
North Carolina State University
Box 8613
Raleigh, NC 27695-8613
(919) 737-3082 (V/TDD)

A federally funded research and training center that works toward improving housing for people with disabilities. Provides technical assistance, training, and publications. Free newsletter, "News," is available in print, large print, computer disk, and cassette.

Department of Housing and Urban Development (HUD)
Special Advisor for Disability Issues
Washington DC 20410-0001
(202) 426-6030 (V/TDD)

Operates programs to make housing accessible, including loans for developers of independent living and group homes and loan and mortgage insurance for rehabilitation of single or multifamily units. Free information kit. Publishes "Adaptable Housing," which offers general and technical information on accessible housing, $3.00; "Fair Housing Amendments Act of 1988: A Selected Resource Guide," $3.00; and a newsletter, "Recent Research Results," free. HUD publications are available from HUD USER (800) 245-2691; in MD, (301) 251-5154.

Electronics Industries Foundation (EIF)
Rehabilitation Engineering Center
1901 Pennsylvania Avenue, NW, Suite 700
Washington DC 20006
(202) 955-5823

A federally funded center that conducts studies related to rehabilitation and financing the equipment needed by people with disabilities. Findings of their research projects are available in manuscript form.

Hyper-ABLEDATA
Trace Research and Development Center
Waisman Center
1500 Highland Avenue
Madison, WI 53705-2280
(608) 262-6966

Assistive technology products are listed in this microcomputer-based version of ABLEDATA (see listing above). Contact Center for hardware requirements and prices.

National Association of Home Builders (NAHB)
National Research Center, Economics and Policy Analysis Division
400 Prince George's Boulevard
Upper Marlboro, MD 20772-8731
(301) 249-4000

The research section of the home building industry trade organization produces publications and provides training on housing and special needs. "Homes for a Lifetime" provides an accessibility checklist, suggest financing alternatives, and recommendations for working with builders and remodelers, $3.00.

VA Office of Technology Transfer
Prosthetics R&D Center
103 South Gay Street
Baltimore, MD 21202
(301) 962-1800

Sponsors rehabilitation research and development of assistive technology. Publishes "Journal of Rehabilitation Research and Development" (see "PUBLICATIONS AND TAPES" section below). The VA Rehabilitation Database includes abstracts of articles in the "Journal of Rehabilitation Research and Development," a section on wheelchairs for adults, adaptive automotive equipment, and information on other assistive devices. The database is available through CompuServe, a subscription computer network. Call Dori Grasso at the number listed above for help or for free introductory time on CompuServe.

<u>Accent on Living</u>
PO Box 700
Bloomington, IL 61702

A magazine with articles, product information, and tips on everyday living. Subscription, one year $8.00; two years, $12.00; add $1.50 for Canada. Also publishes "Accent on Living Buyer's Guide," $10.00.

<u>Adaptable Dwellings</u>
HUD USER
PO Box 6091
Rockville, MD 20850
(800) 245-2691   In Washington DC area, (301) 251-5154

Presents the findings of a research study of the perceptions individuals with disabilities and those without disabilities have toward a variety of adaptations and recommendations that emanated from the study. $8.00

<u>A Consumer's Guide to Home Adaptation</u>
The Adaptive Environments Center
374 Congress Street, Suite 301
Boston, MA 02210
(617) 695-1225 (V/TDD)

A workbook that enables people with disabilities to plan the modifications necessary to adapt their homes. Describes how to widen doorways, lower countertops, etc. $9.50

<u>Directory of On-Line Networks, Databases and Bulletin Boards on Assistive Technology</u>
RESNA Technical Assistance Project
1101 Connecticut Avenue, NW, Suite 700
Washington, DC 20036
(202) 857-1140

Lists public and private organizations which provide information on technology-related services and products through computer networks, databases, and bulletin boards. Free

The Do-Able Renewable Home
by John P. S. Salmen
American Association of Retired Persons (AARP)
Consumer Affairs-Program Department
1909 K Street, NW
Washington, DC 20049
(202) 872-4700

Describes how individuals with disabilities can modify their homes for independent living. Room-by-room modifications are accompanied by illustrations. Free

Eighty-Eight Easy-To-Make Aids for Older People
by Don Caston
Hartley & Marks, Publishers
Box 147
Point Roberts, WA 98281
(206) 945-2017

Practical adaptations for the home with step-by-step instructions. These suggestions would be useful to many individuals with disabilities, regardless of age. $11.95, plus $1.50 postage and handling.

Enabling Products: A Sourcebook
by M. W. Selvidge, M. A. Wylde, and M. Rumage
Institute for Technology Development
Advanced Living Systems Division
428 North Lamar Boulevard
Oxford, MS 38655
(601) 234-0158

A directory of building and household products for people with functional limitations. $35.00

The First Whole Rehab Catalog
by A. Jay Abrams and Margaret Ann Abrams
Betterway Publications, Inc.
PO Box 219
Crozet, VA 22932
(804) 823-5661

Describes adaptive aids and products for independent living. $16.95

Guide to Independent Living for People with Arthritis
Arthritis Foundation
1314 Spring Street, NW
Atlanta, GA 30309
(800) 283-7800   (404) 872-7100

Describes self-help aids, product manufacturers, distributors, and mail order firms. Includes categories such as posture and transfer, mobility aids, grooming, dressing, eating aids, meal preparation, sewing and needlework, communications aids, recreation and leisure, service groups, and funding sources. Illustrated with photographs and drawings. Available through local affiliates of the Arthritis Foundation only; call the Foundation's National Office to request information on your local affiliate.

Independent Living
Public Affairs Directorate
Health & Welfare Canada
Ottawa, Ontario K1A 1B5 Canada

A free series of pamphlets on independent living; includes food preparation, appliances, reaching aids, bathroom equipment and bathing aids, and lifting aids.

Journal of Rehabilitation Research and Development (JRRD)
Office of Technology Transfer
VA Prosthetics R&D Center
103 South Gay Street
Baltimore, MD 21202

A quarterly publication of scientific and engineering articles related to spinal cord injury, prosthetics and orthotics, sensory aids, and gerontology. Includes abstracts of literature, book reviews, and calendar of events. For sale by U.S. Superintendent of Documents, Government Printing Office, Washington DC 20402

Marketplace
Add-Tech
Seaside Education Associates, Inc.
PO Box 341
Lincoln Center, MA 01773
(800) 875-7990

Monthly newsletter which highlights products for everyday living. Free

Tools for Independent Living and Designs for Independent Living
Appliance Information Service (AIS)
Whirlpool Corporation
Administrative Center
Benton Harbor, MI 49022

Provide information on adaptations for the home environment and major appliances. Free

Universal Design: Housing for the Lifespan of All People
Department of Housing and Urban Development (HUD)
Office of Public Affairs
Washington, DC 20410-0050

This brochure describes a universal design concept which makes housing accessible to all individuals regardless of age, size, or ability. No-cost and low-cost options are discussed. Free

Your Home, Your Choice: A Workbook for Older People and Their Families
American Association of Retired Persons (AARP)
Consumer Affairs-Program Department
1909 K Street, NW
Washington, DC 20049
(202) 872-4700

Provides checklists for assessing the home and describes supportive housing alternatives such as housesharing, congregate housing, and retirement homes. Free

ASSISTIVE DEVICES

The following vendors sell assistive devices that help people remain independent. Those that specialize in a specific type of product have a notation under the listing. Otherwise, their product line is broad, usually including personal, health care, and recreation aids, and devices for the home. Unless otherwise noted, the catalogues are free.

ABLEWARE
Maddak, Inc.
661 Route 23
Wayne, NJ 07470
(800) 443-4926   (201) 628-7600

Access to Recreation: Adaptive Recreation Equipment for the Physically Challenged
2509 E. Thousand Oaks Boulevard, Suite 430
Thousand Oaks, CA 91362
(800) 634-4351   (805) 498-7535

Products include exercise equipment and adaptive aids for sports, environmental access, games, hobbies, and crafts.

Access With Ease
PO Box 1150
Chino Valley, AZ 86323
(602) 636-9469

Accessories to Daily Living
Kentel Associates
PO Box 549
Islip, NY 11751-0549
(800) 645-5272

Adaptability
Department 2082
Norwich Avenue
Colchester, CT 06415
(800) 243-9232

Cleo, Inc.
3957 Mayfield Road
Cleveland, OH 44121
(800) 321-0595   (216) 382-9700

Independent Living Aids, Inc.
27 East Mall
Plainview, NY 11803
(800) 537-2118   (516) 752-8080

Maxi-Aids
42 Executive Boulevard
PO Box 3209
Farmingdale, NY 11735
(800) 522-6294   (516) 752-0521

The catalogue is also available as a cassette edition, $2.50, refundable as a coupon with purchase of $25.00 or more. Order #54000.

Medic Alert
PO Box 1009
Turlock, CA 95380
(800) 432-5378

Medical identification bracelet for individuals with serious health conditions.

Radio Shack/Tandy Corporation
500 One Tandy Center
Fort Worth, TX 76102
(817) 390-3700

Radio Shack catalogues include special products for individuals with disabilities such as talking watches and clocks, assistive listening aids, etc.

Sears Home Health Care Catalog
Sears, Roebuck and Co.
Sears Tower
Chicago, IL 60607
(800) 326-1750

Vis-Aids
102-09 Jamaica Avenue
Richmond Hill, NY 11418
(800) 346-9579   (718) 847-4734

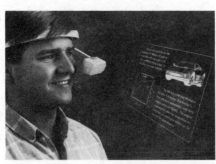
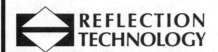
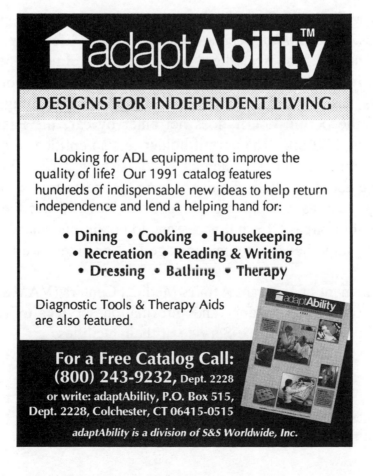

Travel and recreation opportunities for people with disabilities or chronic conditions have expanded greatly in recent years. In the United States and Canada, many state and provincial tourism offices will provide information about accessible attractions for prospective visitors with disabilities. Auto clubs both here and abroad are also good sources for such information.

The Americans with Disabilities Act (ADA) of 1990 requires that fixed route buses and rail transportation be accessible and usable by individuals with disabilities. However, deadlines for implementation of the ADA's regulations vary from six to seven years for private intercity transit to as long as 20 years for Amtrak and commuter rail stations.

The Federal Aviation Administration requires each airline to submit a company-wide policy for travelers with disabilities. Passengers may call ahead to request early boarding, special seating, or meals which meet dietary restrictions. Airport facilities are designed to offer accessible restrooms, elevators, electric carts or wheelchairs, and first aid stations.

Travel agencies that plan special trips for people with disabilities are available throughout the country. Many major hotel chains, airlines, and car rental companies provide special assistance to people with disabilities and often have special toll-free numbers for users of telecommunication devices for the deaf (TDD's). Some companies offer specially trained travel companions to people with disabilities who need an escort.

Individuals with disabilities and elders are eligible for special entrance passes to federal recreation facilities. The *Golden Access Passport* is a free lifetime pass available to any U.S. citizen or permanent resident, regardless of age, who is blind or permanently disabled. It admits the permit holder and passengers in a single, private, noncommercial vehicle to any parks, monuments, historic sites, recreation areas and wildlife refuges which usually charge entrance fees. If the permit holder does not enter by car, the Passport admits the permit holder, spouse, and children. The permit holder is also entitled to a 50 percent discount on charges such as camping, boat launching, and parking fees. Fees charged by private concessionaires are not discounted. Golden Access Passports are available only in person, with proof of disability, such as a certificate of legal blindness. Since the Passport is available at most federal recreation areas, it is not necessary to obtain one ahead of time. A *Golden Age Passport* offers the same benefits to persons aged 62 or older, with proof of age.

Many Department of Veterans Affairs Medical Centers (VAMC) offer driver evaluation services, driving training instruction, and information services to veterans with disabilities through the Rehabilitation Medicine Service at their facilities.

ORGANIZATIONS

(In the listings below, telephone numbers have symbols V for voice and TDD for tele-communication device for the deaf where organizations have published this information.)

Architectural and Transportation Barriers Compliance Board
1111 18th Street NW, Suite 501
Washington, DC 20036-3894
(202) 653-7834

Maintains a database on accessible transportation, including a computerized annotated bibliography. Publishes brochures on subjects such as "Air Carrier Policies on Transport of Battery Powered Wheelchairs."

Association of Driver Educators for the Disabled
c/o ADED Secretariat
33736 La Crosse
Westland, MI 48185
(602) 435-9704

Provides information about training and evaluation facilities for driver education.

Greyhound/Trailways
901 Main Street, Suite 2500
Dallas, TX 75202
(800) 752-4841

The "Helping Hand" Program offers travelers with disabilities the choice of travel with or without a companion. If traveling with a companion who provides assistance, the companion travels free. When traveling alone, if the individual calls Greyhound 24 to 48 hours before departure, the company will arrange for assistance along the route. Travelers with disabilities need not provide proof of disability to qualify for this program. Dog guides for people who are blind, visually impaired, deaf, or hearing impaired may travel at no extra cost. Greyhound/Trailways will carry most types of battery operated wheelchairs, although batteries must be disconnected and stored separately.

MedEscort International, Inc.
ABE International Airport
PO Box 8766
Allentown, PA 18105
(800) 255-7182   (215) 791-3111

Offers specially trained escorts for individuals who cannot travel alone due to age or disability.

Mobility International USA (MIUSA)
PO Box 3551
Eugene, OR 97403
(503) 343-1284 (V/TDD)

Promotes the participation of individuals with disabilities in international and educational exchange programs, such as workcamps, conferences, and student internships. Annual membership, $20.00, includes quarterly newsletter, "Over the Rainbow." Newsletter only, $10.00

National Handicapped Sports
1145 19th Street, NW, Suite 717
Washington, DC 20036
(301) 652-7505   (301) 652-0119 (TDD)

Nationwide network of chapters sponsors recreational activities such as skiing, camping, hiking, biking, horseback riding, and mountain climbing. $15.00 annual membership includes subscription to newsletter, "Handicapped Sport Report."

Society for the Advancement of Travel for the Handicapped (SATH)
26 Court Street
Brooklyn, NY 11242
(718) 858-5483

Provides information on services, publications, and tour operators who specialize in travel arrangements for individuals with disabilities. Annual membership, $40.00; students and people over 65, $25.00.

Travel Information Center
Moss Rehabilitation Hospital
12th and Tabor Road
Philadelphia, PA 19141
(215) 456-9600 (V)   (215) 456-9602 (TDD)

Supplies travel accessibility information about three different locations worldwide for a fee of five dollars.

Travelin' Talk Network
PO Box 3534
Clarksville, TN 37043-3534
(615) 358-2503

Offers information about services and publications for the traveler with a disability. Publishes a newsletter, "Travelin' Talk;" send self-addressed stamped envelope for a free sample.

<u>Wilderness Inquiry</u>
1313 5th Street NE
Minneapolis, MN 55414
(612) 379-3858 (V/TDD)

Sponsors trips into wilderness areas for individuals with disabilities or chronic conditions. Request schedule of current trips.

PUBLICATIONS AND TAPES

<u>Access America: An Atlas and Guide to the National Parks for Visitors with Disabilities</u>
Northern Cartographic
Department BG, PO Box 133
Burlington, VT 05402
(802) 860-2886

Maps of national parks in the U.S. provide information on accessibility of picnic and camping grounds; availability of special communication devices for people with hearing impairments; and availability of trail guides in large print or braille. Special features for readers with vision loss. $89.95; $44.98, individuals or nonprofit organizations; plus $5.00 shipping and handling. Also available: "Access America: A Guide to Yosemite National Park," $7.95. Regional park access guides have been published by Weidenfeld and Nicholson (841 Broadway, New York, NY 10003-4793) and are widely available in local bookstores for $10.95 each.

<u>Access Travel: Airports</u>
S. James
Consumer Information Center L
PO Box 100
Pueblo, CO 81002

A free booklet describing special facilities and services at 519 airports in 62 countries. Order publication 570V.

<u>Air Travel for the Handicapped</u>
Air Transport Association
1709 New York Avenue, NW
Washington, DC 20006
(202) 626-4173

This brochure describes some of the special services available to airline passengers with disabilities. Free

<u>Directory of Travel Agencies for the Disabled</u> $19.95
<u>Travel for the Disabled: A Handbook of Travel Resources and 500 Worldwide Access Guides</u>
$9.95
Twin Peaks Press
PO Box 129
Vancouver, WA 98666-0129
(800) 637-2256   (206) 694-2462

Directory lists travel agents specializing in arrangements for people with disabilities. Handbook provides information about accessibility. Shipping: $2.00 first book, $1.00 additional book.

<u>The Handicapped Driver's Mobility Guide</u>
American Automobile Association (AAA)
Traffic Safety Department
Handicapped Driver Research
1000 AAA Drive
Heathrow, FL 32746
(407) 444-7963

Provides information about adaptive equipment for automobiles, accessories for recreational vehicles and motor homes, driver training, service organizations, and publications for drivers with disabilities. Includes U.S., Canadian, and European resources. $3.00; free to AAA members through local divisions.

<u>Information for Handicapped Travelers</u>
National Library Service for the Blind and Physically Handicapped (NLS)
1291 Taylor Street, NW, Washington DC 20542
(800) 424-8567 or 424-8572

Information about travel agents, transportation, and information centers that specialize in the needs of people with disabilities. Free

<u>Itinerary</u>
PO Box 2012
Bayonne, NJ 07002
(201) 858-3400

Bimonthly newsletter for travelers with disabilities. Includes personal experiences, resources, publications, and health tips for travelers with disabilities. U.S., $10.00; Canada, $13.00

<u>Travel Tips for People with Arthritis</u>
Arthritis Foundation
PO Box 19000
Atlanta, GA 30326
(800) 283-7800   (404) 8772-7100

Advice for individuals who have difficulty walking or who use a cane or wheelchair. Suggestions on selection of accessible hotels, travel agents, and accessible transportation. Free

The Wheelchair Traveler
Accent on Living
PO Box 700
Bloomington, IL 61702
(309) 378-2961

A directory that rates hotels and motels in the United States. $20.00 plus $1.50 shipping

A World of Options for the 1990's: A Guide to International Educational Exchange, Community Service, and Travel for Persons with Disabilities
by Cindy Lewis and Susan Sygall
Mobility International USA (MIUSA)
PO Box 3551
Eugene, OR 97403
(503) 343-1284 (V/TDD)

Lists educational exchange programs, international workcamps, and accessible travel opportunities. Personal experiences are used to describe these programs. Members, $14.00; nonmembers, $16.00.

COMMUNICATION DISORDERS

Because impaired communication can result in social isolation, hearing disorders and speech disorders may have severe effects on individuals. Although speech impairments are sometimes caused by disease, individuals with profound hearing impairments often have speech impairments as well. It is for this reason that both of these communication disorders have been combined into one chapter.

HEARING DISORDERS

Hearing disorders are among the most prevalent conditions resulting in disability in the United States. Although estimates of the number of people with hearing disorders vary widely, there is no doubt that this population is growing. One recent study suggests that nearly eight million Americans age fifteen or older had difficulty hearing a normal conversation, with one-half million completely unable to hear a conversation (U.S. Bureau of the Census: 1986). The National Center for Health Statistics (1988) indicates that the prevalence of deafness and hearing impairments was 21 million during the years 1983 to 1985. Hearing disorders are most common among people age 65 and older. For the general population, the rate was 90.8 per thousand population, and it increased steeply as age increased. For those under 18 years old, the rate was 20.6 per thousand, while for those 75 years or older, the rate was 380.9 per thousand.

Labels such as severe, profound, moderate, and mild hearing impairments have not been clearly defined. Relatively few individuals are totally deaf, unable to perceive any sound whatsoever. People who have severe or profound hearing impairments may be able to hear some sounds, although in large part they are not useful for communication. People who have moderate or mild hearing impairments or who are hard-of-hearing have residual hearing that is useful for communication. Usually these individuals supplement their remaining functional hearing with the use of assistive devices and visual cues.

CAUSES AND TYPES OF HEARING IMPAIRMENT AND DEAFNESS

Congenital hearing disorders may result from viral infections; from the effects of certain drugs taken by the mother during pregnancy; or from problems that occur during labor or delivery. Congenital conditions such as Down's syndrome, cystic fibrosis, and cerebral palsy may also cause hearing loss (Strome: 1989). One type of Usher's syndrome causes congenital deafness, progressive vision loss, and sometimes mental retardation.

Otosclerosis involves the formation of spongy bone, often resulting in the fixation of the ossicles, which are the small bones of the middle ear. This condition can impede the vibrations from passing through this area, thereby causing hearing impairment. Otosclerosis is a progressive disease that often begins in the teenage years or early twenties. Surgery to improve this condition is called stapedectomy; the stapes or stirrup of the middle ear is replaced with a synthetic device capable of vibrating.

Otitis media is an inflammation of the middle ear that is very common in children, although it can occur at any age. Medications usually prevent otitis media from causing permanent hearing loss, but in some cases the inflammation may be chronic, causing permanent damage.

Meningitis is an inflammation of the meninges, which are the membranes that cover the brain and the spinal cord. Hearing loss is sometimes a complication of meningitis, although prompt diagnosis and medication can usually prevent it from occurring.

Hereditary conditions, *trauma*, and the *exposure to loud noise* over a long period of time may also cause hearing impairment. Other possible causes of hearing loss include *stroke* and the *side effects of drugs*, including diuretics used to lower blood pressure and anti-cancer drugs.

There are three major types of hearing loss: conductive, sensorineural, and central. Hearing loss that includes both conductive and sensorineural impairments is referred to as mixed hearing loss.

Conductive hearing loss is an impairment that prevents sound waves from traveling through the outer or middle ear, on the way to the inner ear. This type of impairment reduces the sound, similar to the reduction of sound that results from using ear plugs. Increased amplification of sound enables the person with this type of hearing loss to understand speech in its normal quality (Price and Snider: 1983). Hearing aids are especially effective with this type of hearing loss.

Sensorineural hearing loss results from damage to the cochlea in the inner ear or to the surrounding hair cells that transmit electrical signals to the nerve fibers and the brain. For this reason, many people with this type of hearing impairment are told that they have "nerve deafness." This type of hearing loss is the kind most frequently found in the older population

Tinnitus, considered a sensorineural disorder, is the ringing or buzzing sensation that occurs in the ears in the absence of any external sound. There are a variety of causes for tinnitus, including the use of certain medications. Although there is rarely a cure for tinnitus, there are ways to alleviate its effects. A tinnitus masker substitutes a more acceptable sound for the sound produced by tinnitus. Because hearing loss often accompanies tinnitus, hearing aids are sometimes effective in alleviating the effects. Other treatments that are frequently prescribed are drugs, surgery, biofeedback, and relaxation techniques.

Central hearing loss is the result of damage to nerves in the pathway to the brain or in the brain itself. Although sound levels are not affected, speech discrimination is impaired. Central hearing loss is often a secondary result of other medical conditions, including stroke, head injuries, or vascular problems.

The cochlear implant is a recently developed technique to restore gross hearing function to individuals who are profoundly deaf. Electrodes are implanted to bypass the damaged hair cells surrounding the cochlea. The technique is still in its infancy and is not recommended for most people with hearing loss. It is currently used for selected individuals with profound deafness and, when successful, enables them to hear sounds but not to discriminate speech. Most individuals do not have the profound hearing loss necessary to be considered for this technique (Rupp and Jackson: 1986).

HEARING LOSS IN CHILDREN

One of every 1,000 children is born totally deaf (National Institute on Deafness and Other Communication Disorders: 1989). Congenital hearing loss is usually diagnosed after parents or other care providers have noticed that the child fails to respond to sounds and has not developed speech as expected. Children whose hearing loss is congenital or who experience hearing loss prior to development of language (prelingual) must learn to communicate without the ability to mimic the speech they hear from family members and others. Parents and special teachers for children who are deaf or hearing impaired must help these children to communicate through the use of sign language, speech/lip reading, finger spelling, and oral communication. There is still much to learn about how children who are congenitally deaf or prelingually deaf acquire language and communication skills.

It is essential that children who have hearing impairments be diagnosed early and that intervention begin at once. Sophisticated diagnostic techniques allow the diagnosis of hearing impairments in very small children. Physicians must respond to parents' requests for diagnostic tests and not assume that parents are misguided when they say that their children do not respond to sound. Parents are usually the individuals who have the most knowledge about their child's behavior.

At one time, children who were deaf were forbidden to use sign language or other manual communication, in an effort to integrate them totally into the hearing world; this philosophy is referred to as oral communication or oralism. Today, many advocate "total communication," a philosophy espousing the use of all types of communication methods that enable individuals who are deaf or hearing impaired to communicate with each other as well as with people who have normal hearing.

Most children who are deaf are born to parents with normal hearing. Parents in this situation help their children and themselves by learning alternative means of communication, such as sign language. Sign language has a different structure than oral English. It is a language based on concepts, with the same gesture having several different meanings depending upon its position in relation to the body. Finger spelling, often used in conjunction with sign language, is a system in which each letter of the alphabet is spelled out (Mitchell: 1980). Sign supported speech denotes a communication method using both spoken English and simultaneous signs. Sign supported speech differs from other types of sign languages because it has been specially developed to support the structure and grammar of spoken English. Cued speech is a method that uses hand motions to supplement speechreading. Eight handshapes represent groups of consonant sounds, and four positions about the face represent vowel sounds (Schwartz: 1987). Speech reading, sometimes called lip reading, is a supportive visual process that assists in understanding language. Because many consonants appear as similar mouth shapes, it is impossible to decipher most of spoken English through speech reading alone.

Students who are deaf or hearing impaired are sometimes mainstreamed in regular public school classrooms (See Chapter 3, "Children and Youth" for a discussion of federal laws regarding the education of children with disabilities). How students fare in this environment will depend upon numerous factors, including the onset and severity of the hearing impairment, the student's proficiency in communicating, the support services available, and the knowledge of the school staff in providing appropriate assistance for the student. Teachers in regular classrooms should be educated by vocational rehabilitation professionals, audiologists, or teachers of the deaf about the special needs of students who are deaf or hearing impaired. Teachers should understand that they must face the class when speaking; keep their mouth visible; provide good lighting; let students with hearing impairments sit at the front of the room; and use visual aids whenever possible (Mitchell: 1980). In some cases, it is necessary for an interpreter to be present both in the classroom and during other school activities.

Students who are mainstreamed may encounter problems because they are "different" from their peers. The school years are times when conformity is valued greatly and wearing a hearing aid, speaking differently, or needing an interpreter in the classroom can all present difficult situations for children who are deaf or hearing impaired. Programs to sensitize students to the experience of living with a disability may begin to bring about attitude change and greater acceptance of students who are different. Explaining the nature of the hearing impairment; having students with normal hearing spend time with a simulated hearing loss; and discussing sign language, hearing aids, and the role of interpreters can help to break the ice with classmates. Support services for students who are deaf or hearing impaired include speech and language therapy, audiological services, the services of a classroom aide or interpreter, and environmental adaptations, such as carpeting and acoustical tile.

Students who are interested in pursuing postsecondary education may receive guidance from a vocational or guidance counselor at school or from a rehabilitation counselor at the state vocational rehabilitation department. There are a variety of publications that describe the support services available for students with disabilities at technical institutes, junior colleges, and four year colleges and universities (see "PUBLICATIONS AND TAPES" section below).

Several postsecondary institutions receive federal funding for programs specifically for students who are deaf or hearing impaired (see "ORGANIZATIONS" section below).

A recent report issued by the Commission on Education for the Deaf (1988) concluded that the education of deaf students did not meet acceptable standards. The Commission studied a wide variety of issues, including the availability of elementary, secondary, and postsecondary education and appropriate support services; the qualifications of teachers, audiologists, speech therapists, and interpreters; and the quality of outreach services and research provided by federally funded institutions such as Gallaudet University and the National Technical Institute for the Deaf. Other studies indicate that educational achievements of students who are deaf fall behind their peers with normal hearing (Johnson et al.: 1989).

HEARING LOSS IN ELDERS

As indicated above, hearing loss is most common among people 65 years or older. Most elders experience sensorineural hearing loss, which is not amenable to medical treatment. However, there are many adaptive devices that can help elders cope successfully with hearing loss. The adjustments and psychological effects are much different for people who lose hearing later in life than for those who have congenital or prelingual hearing impairment. For elders, hearing loss is often one of several impairments that they must learn to cope with. A major issue for many elders is acceptance of the fact that they do indeed have a hearing loss. For those elders who live alone, hearing loss may become a threat to safety, as they may be unable to hear a fire alarm or other important alerting devices, such as doorbells. (For a more detailed discussion about hearing loss in elders and services available to help them, see Resources for Elders with Disabilities, described in "PUBLICATIONS AND TAPES" section below.)

PSYCHOLOGICAL ASPECTS OF HEARING LOSS

The effects of hearing impairment and deafness are different for people whose disability occurred congenitally or prelingually than for those whose hearing loss was acquired after they developed speech. Higgins (1980) has described the subculture created by individuals who are prelingually deaf or hearing impaired. These individuals are able to identify with others who have experienced isolation, rejection, and frustration in communications. People who become deaf later in life are audiologically deaf, but not socially deaf, according to Higgins. These individuals are as likely to stigmatize people who are deaf as members of the hearing community.

When a child who is deaf or hearing impaired is born to parents with normal hearing (which is true in the overwhelming number of cases), the amount of change required within the family can be overwhelming. According to Luterman (1987), not only do some parents deny the deafness or hearing impairment for a while, but they may also view the child as fragile. As is often the case when a disabling or chronic condition is present in children, the parents may tend to focus all of their attention on that child to the neglect of their other children. They often must work with a variety of professionals, including physicians, audiologists, and special educators. This process can be very time consuming, resulting in the need to restructure the normal activities of work and home life.

For those individuals whose hearing loss occurred later in life, adjustment in virtually all areas of everyday living is necessary. Tasks that were once taken for granted, such as answering the doorbell or talking on the telephone, now seem to be insurmountable obstacles. As a result, depression is a very common consequence of hearing loss. Studies suggest that people with hearing loss are more likely to be depressed and have low life satisfaction than peers with normal hearing (Glass: 1986). Two factors that frequently undergo change as a result of hearing loss are job satisfaction and relationships with significant others (Weinberger: 1980). Fear of progressive hearing loss and dependency is also a common and natural psychological reaction.

Social withdrawal is another psychological reaction that sometimes accompanies hearing loss. Because some people find it difficult to accept their hearing loss and to seek out appropriate treatment, they try to function as they always did but are unable to do so. Their behavior is often interpreted as mentally inappropriate by family members and friends who are not aware that hearing loss has occurred. In such instances, family members and friends may also withdraw from social encounters. The withdrawal of family and friends reinforces the individual's self-devaluation. In extreme cases, individuals whose hearing loss has not been diagnosed are inappropriately hospitalized for mental disorders.

The ability to hear sound but not to understand words and meanings leads some individuals to believe that speakers are mumbling or speaking too softly. This reaction is often accompanied by a denial that hearing loss has occurred. When individuals deny that they have experienced hearing loss, they will be unwilling to seek assistance from professionals who can provide assistive devices or training to improve their communication. Such a situation often causes frustration for family members and friends of the person with hearing loss and may result in increased tensions within the individual's family setting.

PROFESSIONAL SERVICE PROVIDERS

Otologists are physicians who specialize in diseases of the ear. (Physicians who specialize in treatment of the ear, nose, and throat are called otorhinolaryngologists.) These physicians diagnose and manage diseases that cause hearing problems. For many conditions, medical or surgical treatment results in restoration of hearing. Unfortunately, for most people who experience sensorineural hearing loss, there is no cure. In order to determine if a condition may be improved with medical or surgical intervention, all individuals with hearing loss should be examined by an otologist or otorhinolaryngologist. In cases where there is no effective medical or surgical treatment to restore lost hearing, the physician should refer the patient to an audiologist or a hearing aid dispenser for evaluation for assistive devices.

Audiologists have special training to administer tests to determine the level of functional hearing; to prescribe hearing aids and other devices; to train patients to use the prescribed devices; to refer patients to other professionals and resources; and to train patients in auditory and visual communication (ASHA: 1989). In the case of children, audiologists must work not just with other health care professionals and parents, but also with the school staff to ensure that children have the best assistive devices for the physical setting and that teachers are knowledgeable about the children's needs. Audiologists have either a masters or doctoral degree in audiology and are certified by the American Speech-Language-Hearing Association; in addition, most states license audiologists to practice within the state (Weinstein: 1989). Many audiologists practice in otologists' offices. Others practice in their own private offices, in a hospital or clinic setting, or in a rehabilitation agency.

Hearing aid dispensers sell hearing aids to individuals and are not trained in the diagnosis or treatment of conditions that affect hearing. Some hearing aid dispensers do perform basic audiometric tests. Many individuals are referred to dispensers by audiologists. The U.S. Food and Drug Administration requires a medical evaluation prior to the fitting of hearing aids. Although individuals may sign a waiver that permits hearing aid dispensers to fit a hearing aid without a medical evaluation, it is wise to be examined by a physician to determine whether the condition that is causing the hearing loss may be amenable to medical intervention and whether the underlying condition is causing other medical problems.

Speech therapists may also play a role in the rehabilitation of individuals with hearing loss. Individuals who are congenitally or prelingually deaf or hearing impaired need special training to learn how to speak. Individuals with hearing loss can no longer hear their own voices, so they must learn how to modulate their voices properly. Speech therapists receive certificates of clinical competence (CCC) from the American Speech-Language-Hearing Association.

Teachers of the deaf receive special training in university programs located throughout the country. They receive certification from the Council on Education of the Deaf (See "ORGANIZATIONS" section below). They may work in special schools for the deaf or in public schools. Regular classroom teachers with students who are deaf or hearing impaired in their classes should receive training in techniques that maximize the educational environment for these students.

Interpreters facilitate communication between individuals who are deaf or hearing impaired and individuals with normal hearing who are not fluent in sign language. The interpreter may be viewed as a translator and does not contribute any of his or her own comments to the conversation. The language the interpreter uses should be chosen by the person who is deaf or hearing impaired. It may be American Sign Language; another type of sign language that is correlated with spoken English; or oral interpreting, which uses natural lip movements without speech (Watson: 1990).

Vocational rehabilitation counselors help individuals with hearing disorders prepare for independent living and for job placement. Rehabilitation includes prescription of appropriate assistive devices, training in the use of these devices, training in techniques such as speech-reading or sign language to enhance communication, and counseling for both the individual with hearing loss and family members. Vocational rehabilitation counselors may help to locate the appropriate assistive listening devices necessary to perform the requirements of a specific position and help the employer to modify the environment for individuals who are deaf or hearing impaired.

Since hereditary conditions are responsible for some types of hearing impairment, *genetic counselors* may play an important role. Genetic counselors are specially trained and often work in a multidisciplinary team of physicians, social workers, and nurses. They obtain information about the family's medical history and the pregnancy history of the mother. Audiograms and physical examinations for family members may help the geneticist determine the cause of the hearing impairment. Geneticists are sometimes able to explain the hereditary process by which the genes causing deafness or hearing impairment were passed on to succeeding generations. Knowing whether a hearing impairment is hereditary and the probability of passing it on to offspring can be a valuable asset in family planning.

WHERE TO FIND SERVICES

Many states have special offices to provide services to individuals who are deaf or hearing impaired. These agencies often provide assistive devices, interpreters, vocational counseling, special educational programs, and counseling and advocacy. The specific services and the populations served vary by state. Individuals should contact the state government information operator, the state office serving individuals with disabilities, or the state department of vocational rehabilitation services to determine if an office for people who are deaf or hearing impaired exists in their state. In addition, state offices of vocational rehabilitation provide services for individuals who are deaf or hearing impaired and are interested in retaining their current positions or receiving training for new careers. Some state agencies, private agencies, university programs, and adult education courses teach sign language to family members of individuals who are deaf or hearing impaired.

Local agencies providing services to people who are deaf or hearing impaired include hospitals with otology or otolaryngology departments; private agencies that specialize in services and rehabilitation for individuals who are deaf or hearing impaired; independent living centers; audiologists and otologists in private practice or at speech and hearing clinics; hearing aid dispensers (listed in the Yellow Pages); universities that have graduate programs for audiologists or speech therapists; and Veterans Affairs Medical Centers. Some general rehabilitation facilities provide special rehabilitation for people who are deaf or hearing impaired.

Most children who are totally deaf or profoundly hearing impaired spend at least some time in residential schools for the deaf (Schein and Delk: 1974), which are often state supported institutions. Other educational options for children who are deaf or hearing impaired include special day schools; special classes within a regular school; and mainstreaming in a regular school, with the assistance of a speech therapist, interpreter, classroom aide, or resource room teacher. Local education agencies are required to provide services for children and youth with disabilities (see Chapter 3, "Children and Youth"). Parents may benefit by joining support groups composed of parents of children who are deaf or hearing impaired or other formal organizations that provide counseling and referral for parents.

Public libraries are a good source of directories of local agencies. In addition, some libraries and museums have special programs for people with hearing disorders. An increasing number of performances and social events have special amplification devices available for people with hearing loss. (See "ASSISTIVE DEVICES" section below.)

ENVIRONMENTAL ADAPTATIONS

Most children who are deaf or hearing impaired will receive prescriptions for hearing aids and other assistive devices from audiologists and school personnel. As they move through the school system or change schools, re-evaluation of both hearing aids, other assistive devices, and the environment should be carried out on a regular basis. Those individuals who have congenital disorders are likely to remain stable, but requirements of given tasks may change, creating the need for changes in the adaptive equipment.

It is not uncommon for people with acquired hearing loss to resist the use of adaptive equipment. Meeting with other people who have successfully adapted to the use of hearing aids or other devices may encourage those who are resistant to seek out these devices themselves. Purchasing hearing aids and other devices that include a trial period may also encourage resistant individuals.

People with acquired hearing loss should consider the wide variety of options available to improve their communication skills. For example, they should consider speech-reading, a technique that maximizes visual clues from lip movements and other body gestures as well as learning to think about the context of the speech. Individuals should always face the speaker during a conversation in order to see these visual cues.

Environmental adaptations should also be made at health care providers' offices, hospitals, rehabilitation centers, senior citizen centers, and any facility that is designed for group use, such as theaters, churches, and the like. New buildings and those being renovated should have good acoustics. For example, curtains and carpets absorb background noise (Dion: 1989). Amplification systems and assistive listening devices should be installed.

Family, friends, and service providers should all learn how to communicate effectively with people with hearing loss. The following tips will save much frustration when holding a conversation with someone who is deaf or hearing impaired:

- Be certain that the person knows that you are speaking to him or her.

- Always face the person throughout the conversation so that he or she may get visual cues. Be certain that your mouth is visible throughout the conversation, even if the person with hearing loss is not an experienced lip reader.

- Be certain that background noises have been eliminated. For example, radios, televisions, and the like should not be playing and water should not be running.

- Speak clearly at a level just slightly above normal, but do not shout.

- If the person does not understand what you are saying, rephrase the sentence.

- Ask the person if he or she has understood you.

- When speaking to a person through an interpreter, look directly at the person and speak in the same way as you would in any other conversation. Do not say to the interpreter, "Ask him or her..."

ASSISTIVE DEVICES

The types of devices most appropriate to a given individual depend upon not only the type and severity of the hearing impairment but also the individual's usual activities. The variety of assistive devices available to help people with hearing loss communicate effectively is constantly expanding. Major organizations such as SHHH, ASHA, and the National Information Center on Deafness at Gallaudet University (See "ORGANIZATIONS" section below) publish information about a wide range of devices. For those individuals who are not able to afford the devices they need, financial assistance is often available through a state agency or through local service organizations. Assistive devices are available on display at local rehabilitation agencies.

The most common device, the *hearing aid*, has undergone considerable improvement in recent years, and there are many types and models to choose from. The reluctance on the part of many people to use hearing aids may be attributed in part to denial of hearing loss, the high cost of some hearing aids, the failure of many medical insurance policies to cover the cost, and improper training in the use of hearing aids.

Because hearing aids amplify sound, they amplify background noises as well as conversation. The amplification of background noise is a common reason that some people do not find hearing aids useful. Some hearing aids are designed to screen out certain frequencies and background noises; however, no model is capable of enhancing speech and eliminating background noise perfectly. Experts recommend that people with hearing loss purchase hearing aids with a 30 day trial period, so they may be returned or adjusted if not satisfactory. Because the level of hearing impairment may change, individuals should be re-evaluated on a regular basis and whenever a decrease in hearing ability is noticed.

Assistive listening devices (ALD's) are alternative devices for situations where hearing aids are not sufficient. ALD's transmit sound waves directly into the ears of people with hearing loss. They utilize microphones close to the source of the sound, amplifiers, and headsets. Three types of ALD's are infrared, FM, and hard-wired systems. The first two types of systems are useful in group situations and are currently available in large group settings such as theaters and churches, while the hard-wired system is often useful in the home situation and may be installed inexpensively (Weinstein: 1989).

Telecommunication devices for the deaf (TDD's) transmit printed messages across telephone lines. They utilize computers with screens and keyboards as well as a modem, which serves as the communication device. In some states, the agency serving individuals who are deaf or hearing impaired or the vocational rehabilitation agency provides TDD's free on loan or offers them for sale at a discount price. TDD's may only be used when there is a TDD at the other end of the telephone line. However, some telephone companies offer a relay service when one party does not have a TDD. The Americans with Disabilities Act mandates that telephone companies provide 24 hour relay services so that individuals who have TDD's may communicate with individuals who do not have TDD's (beginning July 26, 1993). Telephone companies can provide information about installing a TDD. A TDD operator is available (800-855-1155) for directory assistance and placing credit card, collect, person-to-person and third party calls.

Hand-held *telephone amplifiers* and *volume controls* are available to attach to phones at home and are useful when traveling. These devices have become so commonplace that many stores and mail order catalogues that sell phone equipment stock amplifiers as well as TDD's.

Visual alerting systems are available to use as smoke or fire detectors and as indicators that the telephone or doorbell is ringing. *Vibrators* are available to substitute for an audible signal from an alarm clark.

Hearing ear dogs are used in ways that are similar to guide dogs for people with vision impairments. Dogs are trained to lead their owners to the source of sound and enable people with hearing loss, especially those who live alone, to maintain their independence and security.

Closed captioned television programs, which were relatively rare just a few years ago, are becoming more common, with all major network programs in prime time now closed captioned. Closed captioning provides a print output of the program's speech at the bottom of the television screen. Closed captioned programs are accessible through decoders, which are available through a variety of outlets and cost about two-hundred dollars or less. The Television Decoder Circuitry Act (PL 101-431) mandates that all television sets with screens 13 inches or larger for sale after July 1, 1993 be manufactured with built-in decoders for closed captions. Many videotaped movies available for rental or purchase are also close-captioned.

References

Champagne, J.R. and B. Dion
1983 <u>Building Performance for the Hearing Impaired</u> paper delivered at Toronto Conference, "A Sound Beginning" cited in Betty Dion, "Designing a Barrier-Free Environment" <u>Rehabilitation Digest</u> Spring, 1989

Commission on Education of the Deaf
1988 <u>Toward Equality</u> A Report to the President and the Congress of the United States Washington D.C.: U.S. Government Printing Office

Dion, Betty
1989 "Designing a Barrier-Free Environment" <u>Rehabilitation Digest</u> (Spring):12-14

Fein, D.J.
1983 "Projection of Speech and Hearing Impairments to 2050" <u>ASHA</u> 25(November):31

Glass, Laurel E.
1986 "Rehabilitation for Deaf and Hearing-Impaired Elderly" pp. 218-236 in Stanley J. Brody and George E. Ruff (eds.) <u>Aging and Rehabilitation</u> New York: Springer

Higgins, Paul C.
1980 <u>Outsiders in a Hearing World</u> Beverly Hills, CA: Sage Publications

Johnson, Robert E., Scott K. Liddell, and Carol J. Erting
1989 <u>Unlocking the Curriculum: Principles for Achieving Access in Deaf Education</u> Washington D.C.: Gallaudet Research Institute

Luterman, David
1987 <u>Deafness in the Family</u> Boston: Little Brown, College Hill Publications

Mitchell, Joyce Slayton
1980 <u>See Me More Clearly</u> New York: Harcourt, Brace, Jovanovich

National Center for Health Statistics, John Gary Collins
1988 "Prevalence of Selected Chronic Conditions, United States, 1983-1985" <u>Advance Data From Vital and Health Statistics</u>, No. 155 DHHS Pub. No. (PHS) 88-1250 Public Health Service, Hyattsville, MD

National Institute on Deafness and Other Communication Disorders
1989 <u>National Strategic Research Plan</u> Bethesda, MD: National Institutes of Health

Price, Lloyd L. and Robert M. Snider
1983 "The Geriatric Patient: Ear, Nose and Throat Problems" in William Reichel (ed.) <u>Clinical Aspects of Aging</u> Baltimore, MD: Williams and Wilkins

Rupp, Ralph R. and Patricia D. Jackson
1986 "Primary Care for the Hearing Impaired: A Changing Picture" <u>Geriatrics</u> 41(March):75-80

Schein, Jerome D. and Marcus T. Delk, Jr.
1974 <u>The Deaf Population of the United States</u> Silver Spring, MD: National Association of the Deaf

Strome, Marshall
1989 "Hearing Loss and Hearing Aids" <u>Harvard Medical School Health Letter</u> 14(April):6:5-8

U.S. Bureau of the Census
1986 <u>Disability, Functional Limitation, and Health Insurance Coverage: 1984/85</u> Current Population Reports, Series P-70, No. 8, Washington, DC: U.S. Government Printing Office

Weinberger, Morris
1980 "Social and Psychological Consequences of Legitimating a Hearing Impairment" <u>Social Science and Medicine</u> 14A:213-222

Weinstein, Barbara
1989 "Geriatric Hearing Loss: Myths, Realities, Resources for Physicians" <u>Geriatrics</u> 44(April):42-59

ORGANIZATIONS

(In the listings below, telephone numbers have symbols V for voice and TDD for tele-communication device for the deaf where organizations have published this information.)

Alexander Graham Bell Association for the Deaf
3417 Volta Place, NW
Washington DC 20007-2778
(202) 337-5220 (V/TDD)

A membership organization that provides services and support for people who are deaf or hearing impaired. Sponsors conferences and workshops. Special section for parents of children who are deaf or hearing impaired and special publications addressing children's needs. Publishes "Volta Review," a professional journal, and "Newsounds," a newsletter; both included with membership. Regular membership, $40.00

American Deafness and Rehabilitation Association (ADARA)
Box 55369
Little Rock, AR 72225
(501) 375-6643 (V/TDD)

An interdisciplinary organization for both professionals and consumers. Promotes development of services to people who are deaf or hearing impaired. Publishes "Journal of American Deafness and Rehabilitation Association" with research findings and "ADARA Newsletter." Regular membership, $43.00

American Society for Deaf Children (ASDC)
814 Thayer Avenue
Silver Spring, MD 20910
(301) 585-5400   (301) 585-5401 (TDD)

A membership organization for parents of children who are deaf, ASDC provides resource materials, makes referrals, and holds a biennial meeting. Newsletter, "Endeavor," published six times per year; free with membership. Individual/family membership, $25.00

American Speech-Language-Hearing Association (ASHA)
10801 Rockville Pike
Rockville, MD 20852
(800) 638-8255   (301) 897-5700 (V/TDD)

A professional organization of speech and language pathologists and audiologists. Provides information on hearing aids and communication problems and a free list of certified audiologists and speech therapists for each state.

American Tinnitus Association
PO Box 5
Portland, OR 97207
(503) 248-9985

Membership organization that carries out and supports research and education on tinnitus and other ear diseases. Provides resources to both professionals and patients about seeking help and information. Also provides cassette tapes of environmental sounds that may provide relief from tinnitus. Self-help groups for members. Basic membership fee, $15.00

Architectural and Transportation Barriers Compliance Board
1111 18th Street, NW, Suite 501
Washington DC 20036-3894
(800) 872-2253 (V/TDD)   (202) 653-7834 (V/TDD)

A federal agency charged with setting federal standards for accessibility and assisting federal personnel and others in carrying out federal laws. Provides technical assistance, sponsors research, and distributes publications.

Arkansas Rehabilitation Research and Training Center on Deafness and Hearing Impairment
4601 West Markham Street
Little Rock, AR 72205
(501) 371-1654

A federally funded research center which focuses on enhancing the transition from school to work for people who are deaf or hearing impaired. Also addresses communication and adjustment skills. Sponsors workshops, conferences, and graduate training programs.

Association of Late-Deafened Adults (ALDA)
PO Box 641763
Chicago, IL 60664-1763

Sponsors a network of self-help groups for adults throughout the United States and Canada who experienced hearing loss as adults. Provides information and consultations for professionals and the public. Publishes newsletter, "ALDA News." Operates ALDA TDD Online, which provides national and local (Chicago) news, 24 hours a day, every day of the year [(312) 604-4192]. Individual membership, $12.00; professional/organization membership, $30.00

Better Hearing Institute
Box 1840
Washington, DC 20013
(800) 327-9355   (703) 642-0580

Provides information about hearing loss, available treatments, and dispensers.

Canadian Hearing Society
271 Spadina Road, Room 311
Toronto, Ontario M5R 2V3 Canada
(416) 964-9595 (V)   (416) 964-0023 (TDD)

Provides direct services including screening for hearing loss, counseling, hearing aids, technical devices, and information services. Advocates on behalf of hearing impaired and deaf individuals. Main office in Toronto with regional offices throughout Canada.

Council for Exceptional Children (CEC)
1920 Association Drive
Reston, VA 22091
(703) 620-3660

A professional membership organization that works toward improving the quality of education for children who have disabilities or are gifted; special division for communication disorders. Regular membership, $55.00

Council on Education of the Deaf
c/o Committee on Professional Preparation and Certification
Gallaudet University
800 Florida Avenue, NE
Washington DC 20002

Sets standards for certification for educators of the deaf and accredits university training programs.

The Education and Auditory Research (EAR) Foundation
2000 Church Street, Box 111
Nashville, TN 37236
(800) 545-4327   (615) 329-7809 (V/TDD)

Provides public information about hearing disorders and operates a hearing ear dog program. Request catalogue of professional education programs, reprints of scientific articles, and videotapes.

Gallaudet Research Institute (GRI)
Gallaudet University
800 Florida Avenue, NE
Washington DC 20002
(202) 651-5714 (V/TDD)

Conducts research on all aspects of deafness and hearing impairment. Newsletter, "Research at Gallaudet," reviews research findings. Free

Gallaudet University
800 Florida Avenue, NE
Washington DC 20002
202) 651-5000 (V/TDD)

The recipient of federal funding, Gallaudet is a university for deaf students with special model educational programs for students in elementary and secondary school. Classes are taught in sign language, and a wide range of support services are available. Conducts outreach programs through distribution of educational materials developed at Gallaudet, workshops, seminars, and consultations with school departments throughout the country.

Helen Keller National Center for Deaf-Blind Youths and Adults
111 Middle Neck Road
Sands Point, NY 11050
(516) 944-8900 (V/TDD)

Provides evaluation for rehabilitation through regional field offices throughout U.S. Publishes "National Center News," free.

House Ear Institute (HEI)
2100 West Third Street
Los Angeles, CA 90057
(213) 483-4431   (213) 484-2642

Studies the causes of hearing impairments and trains professionals in diagnosis, treatment, and rehabilitation. Publishes newsletter, "Oto Review." Free catalogue of audio-visual materials.

National Association of the Deaf (NAD)
814 Thayer Avenue
Silver Spring, MD 20910
(301) 587-1788 (V/TDD)

A membership organization with state chapters throughout the U.S. Advocates for its members and serves as an information clearinghouse. Members receive a newspaper, "The Broadcaster," and a magazine, the "Deaf American," plus a 20% discount on NAD publications. Special programs for youth and special sections for senior citizens, federal employees, and sign instructors. Holds national and regional conventions. Individual membership, $25.00. Free catalogue of publications.

National Captioning Institute
5203 Leesburg Pike
Falls Church, VA 22041
(800) 533-9673 (V)   (800) 321-8337 (TDD)   (703) 998-2400 (V/TDD)

Provides closed-captioning for television programs and videotapes. Distributes TeleCaption decoders to retail outlets. Call toll-free number to obtain distributor in your location.

National Center for Law and the Deaf
Gallaudet University
800 Florida Avenue, NE
Washington DC 20002
(202) 651-5373 (V/TDD)

Handles cases involving consumer and employment discrimination related to deafness. Answers individual telephone inquiries.

National Information Center on Deafness (NICD)
Gallaudet University
800 Florida Avenue, NE
Washington, DC 20002
(202) 651-5051 (V)   (202) 651-5052 (TDD)

Provides information on a wide variety of topics related to deafness and hearing loss. Makes referrals to local and community services. Free catalogue of publications.

National Institute on Deafness and Other Communication Disorders
National Institutes of Health
Building 31, Room 1B-62
9000 Rockville Pike
Bethesda, MD 20892
(301) 496-7243   (301) 492-0252 (TDD)

Federal agency that funds basic research studies on problems of hearing, balance, voice, language, and speech.

National Technical Institute for the Deaf (NTID)
Rochester Institute of Technology
Lomb Memorial Drive, PO Box 9887
Rochester, NY 14623
(716) 475-6824 (V/TDD)

A federally funded technical college created for deaf students within a larger institution for students with normal hearing. Students may enroll in courses in the other colleges within the Rochester Institute of Technology.

Registry of Interpreters for the Deaf (RID)
8719 Colesville Road, Suite 310
Silver Spring, MD 20910
(301) 608-0050 (V/TDD)

The national certifying organization for interpreters. Establishes guidelines for professional interpreters. Produces guide of training programs for interpreters throughout the country. Maintains a list of interpreters and postsecondary institutions that offer interpreter training programs.

Rehabilitation Engineering Center for Technological Aids for Deaf and Hearing Impaired Individuals
The Lexington Center
30th Avenue and 75th Street
Jackson Heights, NY 11370
(718) 899-8800

A federally funded center that conducts research into hearing aid technology and alternate technologies.

Self Help for Hard of Hearing People (SHHH)
7800 Wisconsin Avenue
Bethesda, MD 20814
(301) 657-2248 (V)   (301) 657-2249 (TDD)

National membership organization with local and regional chapters. Provides information, support, and individual referrals. Membership, U.S., $15.00; Canada, $20.00; includes subscription to bimonthly magazine "SHHH" and a discount on many publications.

Telecommunications for the Deaf
814 Thayer Avenue
Silver Spring, MD 20910
(301) 589-3786 (V)   (301) 589-3006 (TDD)

Membership organization that lobbies for improved telecommunication for individuals who deaf or hearing impaired. Publishes "International Directory of TDD Users" annually. Individual membership, $15.00; business/organization membership, $30.00; includes directory listing and copy of directory as well as newsletter, "GA-SK."

Tripod
2901 North Keystone Street
Burbank, CA 91504
(800) 352-8888 (V/TDD)   In CA, (800) 346-8888 (V/TDD)
(818) 972-2080 (V/TDD)

A support and referral service for parents of children who are deaf or hearing impaired. Hotline will respond to individual questions. Produces educational brochures and videotapes to help parents learn how to interact with children who are deaf.

University of California San Francisco Center on Deafness
3333 California Street, Suite 10
San Francisco, CA 94143-1208
(415) 476-4980   (415) 476-7600 (TDD)

A federally funded research and training center that focuses on the mental health needs of people who are deaf. Sponsors conferences and graduate training. Articles available documenting findings of research projects. Publishes "UCCD Newsletter."

U.S. Department of Veterans Affairs (VA)
Prosthetics Division, local VA Medical Centers

Provides free hearing aids to eligible veterans and Tele-Caption decoder for veterans with hearing loss that is service related.

VA Office of Technology Transfer
Prosthetics R&D Center
103 South Gay Street
Baltimore, MD 21202
(301) 962-1800

Sponsors rehabilitation research and development of assistive technology. Publishes "Journal of Rehabilitation Research and Development" (see "PUBLICATIONS AND TAPES" section below). The VA Rehabilitation Database includes abstracts of articles in the "Journal of Rehabilitation Research and Development" and a section on assistive hearing devices. The database is available through CompuServe, a subscription computer network. Call Dori Grasso at the number listed above for help or for free introductory time on CompuServe.

(Publications focusing specifically on assistive devices are listed under "RESOURCES FOR ASSISTIVE DEVICES" below.)

American Annals of the Deaf Reference Issue
Pre-College Outreach Program
Gallaudet University
KDES, PAS-6
800 Florida Avenue, NE
Washington DC 20002-3625

The annual reference issue is published each spring and lists special schools and programs throughout the United States and Canada. $22.50

Choices in Deafness: A Parents Guide
by Sue Schwartz
Woodbine House
10400 Connecticut Avenue
Kensington, MD 20895
(800) 843-7323

Discusses the various services children who are deaf or hearing impaired need; the choices in communication; and case studies of parents and children who have successfully adapted to deafness or hearing impairment. $12.95

College and Career Programs for Deaf Students
Center for Assessment and Demographic Studies
Gallaudet University
800 Florida Avenue, NE
Washington DC 20002

Describes admissions, costs, degrees available, and support services for deaf students at postsecondary programs throughout the United States and Canada. $12.95 plus $1.50 postage

Coping with Hearing Loss
by Susan V. Rezen and Carl Hausman
Dembner Books
80 Eighth Avenue
New York, NY 10011

Discusses causes of hearing loss, problems experienced by people with hearing loss, solutions for these problems, information about hearing aids, and tips on speechreading. $15.95

Facilitating the Transition of Deaf Adolescents to Adulthood
Arkansas Rehabilitation Research and Training Center on Deafness and Hearing Impairment
4601 West Markham Street
Little Rock, AR 72205
(501) 371-1654

Discusses how parents and professionals can work together to help adolescents and what rehabilitation counselors can do for this age group. $15.00

Growing Together
National Information Center on Deafness
Gallaudet University
800 Florida Avenue, NE
Washington, DC 20002
(202) 651-5051 (V)   (202) 651-5052 (TDD)

A publication that answers the questions commonly asked by parents of children who are deaf or hearing impaired. Addresses acceptance, communication, and educational issues. $7.00

How the Student with Hearing Loss Can Succeed in College
by Carol Flexer, Denise Wray, and Ron Leavitt
Alexander Graham Bell Association for the Deaf
3417 Volta Place, NW
Washington DC 20007-2778
(202) 337-5220 (V/TDD)

Provides information for students who plan to attend universities. Includes information about support services, financial aid, and technological services. $18.95 plus $3.00 shipping

Journal of Rehabilitation Research and Development (JRRD)
Office of Technology Transfer
VA Prosthetics R&D Center
103 South Gay Street
Baltimore, MD 21202

A quarterly publication of scientific and engineering articles including those related to sensory aids and gerontology. Includes abstracts of literature, book reviews, and calendar of events. For sale by U.S. Superintendent of Documents, Government Printing Office, Washington DC 20402

Legal Rights of Hearing-Impaired People
Gallaudet University Press
800 Florida Avenue, NE
Washington DC 20002
(800) 451-1073 (V/TDD) book orders and information only   (202) 651-5488 (V/TDD)

Discusses the legal rights of people with hearing impairments in situations such as employment, education, and health care. Federal and state statutes included. $13.95

Lipreading Made Easy
Alexander Graham Bell Association for the Deaf
3417 Volta Place, NW
Washington, DC 20007-2778
(202) 337-5220 (V/TDD)

Lessons in how to use vision to accommodate for hearing loss. Print version, $13.95 plus $5.00 shipping and handling; two-hour videotape (VHS) with captions, $75.00 plus $7.00 shipping and handling

Living with Hearing Loss
Resources for Rehabilitation
33 Bedford Street, Suite 19A
Lexington, MA 02173
(617) 862-6455

One title in a series of large print publications designed for distribution by professionals to people with disabilities. Includes information on how to obtain services, organizations that serve people with hearing loss, publications, and aids that help people with hearing loss. Minimum purchase 25 copies. $2.00 per copy. See order form opposite inside back cover.

Meeting the Needs of Employees with Disabilities
Resources for Rehabilitation
33 Bedford Street, Suite 19A
Lexington, MA 02173
(617) 862-6455

Provides information to help people with disabilities retain or obtain employment. Information on government programs and laws, supported employment, training programs, environmental adaptations, and the transition from school to work are included. Chapters on mobility, vision, hearing, and speech impairments include information on organizations, products, and services that enable employers to accommodate the needs of employees with disabilities. $42.95 plus $5.00 shipping and handling

<u>Resources for Elders with Disabilities</u>
Resources for Rehabilitation
33 Bedford Street, Suite 19A
Lexington, MA 02173
(617) 862-6455

A large print resource directory that describes services and products that help elders with disabilities to function independently. Includes chapters on hearing loss, stroke, vision loss, arthritis, diabetes, and osteoporosis. $39.95 plus $5.00 shipping and handling

<u>Students Who are Deaf or Hard of Hearing in Postsecondary Education</u>
HEATH Resource Center
One Dupont Circle, NW, Suite 800
Washington DC 20036-1193
(800) 544-3284 (V/TDD)   (202) 939-9320

A discussion of the various options for students who plan to go on to postsecondary education. Discusses the types of support services available, financial assistance, information for faculty and staff, and helpful publications. Free

RESOURCES FOR ASSISTIVE DEVICES

(Listed below are publications that provide information about assistive devices and catalogues that specialize in devices for people with hearing loss. Generic catalogues that sell some aids for people with hearing loss are listed in Chapter 4, "Making Everyday Living Easier." In the listings below, telephone numbers have symbols V for voice and TDD for telecommunication device for the deaf where organizations have published this information.)

Alerting and Communication Devices for Hearing Impaired People
National Information Center on Deafness
Gallaudet University
800 Florida Avenue, NE
Washington, DC 20002
(202) 651-5051 (V)   (202) 651-5052 (TDD)

A basic guide to the major categories of assistive devices. Single copy, free; multiple copies, $.50 each.

Assistive Devices for Hearing-Impaired Persons
New York League for the Hard of Hearing
71 West 23rd Street
New York, NY 10010-4162
(212) 741-7650 (V)   (212) 255-1932 (TDD)

A videotape demonstrating devices that supplement the use of hearing aids. $75.00 plus $5.00 shipping

AT & T Special Needs Center
2001 Route 46, Suite 310
Parsippany, NJ 07054-9990
(800) 233-1222 (V)   (800) 833-3232 (TDD)

Free catalogue of telephone amplifiers, caption decoders, TDD's, etc.

Financing the Purchase of Devices for Deaf and Severely Hard of Hearing People: A Directory of Sources
Gallaudet Research Institute
Publication Series - Fay House
Gallaudet University
800 Florida Avenue, NE
Washington DC 20002

Provides information about programs that purchase, finance, or lend assistive devices for people who cannot afford to purchase them on their own. $5.50

Food and Drug Administration (FDA)
Office of Consumer Affairs
5600 Fishers Lane
Rockville, MD 20857
(301) 443-3170 (V)   (301) 443-4190 (TDD)

Distributes free publications about hearing aids, which are regulated by the FDA. Write for a list of current titles.

Handyman Hints for Hard of Hearing Helps
Self Help for Hard of Hearing People (SHHH)
7800 Wisconsin Avenue
Bethesda, MD 20814
(301) 657-2248 (V)   (301) 657-2249 (TDD)

Do-it-yourself tips on creating economical assistive listening devices. Members, $6.00; nonmembers, $8.00

Hear You Are Inc.
4 Musconetcong Avenue
Stanhope, NJ 07874
(201) 347-7662

Free catalogue of phone devices, caption decoders, etc.

National Catalog House of the Deaf
4300 North Kilpatrick Avenue
Chicago, IL 60641
(312) 283-2907 (V)   (312) 736-6243 (TDD)

Free catalogue of a variety of devices including TDD's, caption decoders, alerting systems, etc.

Specialized Audio, Visual, and Tactile Alerting Devices for Deaf and Hard of Hearing People
Gallaudet Research Institute
Publication Series - Fay House
Gallaudet University
800 Florida Avenue, NE
Washington DC 20002

Describes assistive devices including alerting systems, telephone devices, pagers, etc. $3.50

Telecommunications Devices for the Deaf: A Guide to Selection, Ordering, and Installation
Architectural and Transportation Barriers Compliance Board
1111 18th Street, NW, Suite 501
Washington DC 20036-3894
(202) 653-7834 (V/TDD)

A brochure with basic information about TDD's. The Architectural and Transportation Barriers Compliance Board offers technical assistance on TDD's. Free

What You Should Know about TDDs
National Technical Institute for the Deaf
Rochester Institute of Technology
Lomb Memorial Drive, PO Box 9887
Rochester, NY 14623
(716) 475-6824 (V/TDD)

Free publication (limit 10 copies) with information about telecommunication devices for the deaf.

SPEECH DISORDERS

Over 2.5 million Americans over the age of 15 have difficulty having their speech understood. This disability affects 1% of the population age 15 to 64 years and 3.5% of the population 65 years or over (U.S. Bureau of the Census: 1986). The inability to communicate effectively creates a barrier to all types of social interactions, including education and employment.

CAUSES AND TYPES OF SPEECH IMPAIRMENTS

There are four types of speech impairments. *Disorders of articulation* include omission, distortion, substitution, or addition of sounds. These disorders may be either functional with no known organic cause, or they may have organic origins, such as cerebral palsy, brain damage, or cleft palate (Goldenson: 1978). *Disorders of the voice* involve defects of pitch and volume. These disorders are sometimes caused by abnormal growths on the vocal cords or by hearing impairments.

Disorders of time and rhythm of sound production result in speech that is difficult to listen to and is sometimes unintelligible. Stuttering is the most common type of disorder of time and rhythm. Stuttering is an involuntary hesitation in producing sounds or an involuntary repetition of the same sound. About 2.5 million Americans, or one percent of the population, stutter (Fraser: 1990). The cause of stuttering is unknown, although it has often been attributed to psychological problems.

Aphasia or *dysphasia* is the inability to recognize and use symbols and expressions. There are many different types of aphasia. Some individuals with aphasia are able to speak fluently, but their understanding of speech is impaired. Others comprehend written and oral language but are nonfluent. Still others have difficulty in seeking appropriate words and occasionally substitute words or letters. In global aphasia, all aspects of speech and language are impaired (Albert and Helm-Estabrooks: 1988). In most cases, aphasia is caused by a stroke, but brain tumors and head injury may also cause aphasia.

As noted above, many speech impairments are the result of *deafness or severe hearing impairment*. Teaching speech to children who are congenitally or prelingually deaf is a slow, laborious process. Visual cues help children to understand conversations. The delay in acquisition of language may affect the child's ability to keep pace with standard educational objectives. The individual never develops the same speaking skills that individuals with normal hearing do (Bowe: 1978). Deaf children have different articulation, frequency, and voice quality patterns than hearing children (Bernstein et al.: 1990).

Cancer of the larynx is another cause of speech impairment. In advanced stages of the disease, the larynx, which contains the vocal cords, is removed surgically. Individuals whose larynx has been removed (often referred to as laryngectomees) must learn new ways of speaking, or they may use an artificial larynx. Artificial larynxes enable an early return to work while speech training is taking place; they also enable individuals whose surgery has been extensive or who do not have the motivation to learn a new way of speaking to continue oral communication.

Esophageal speech is a method that uses belches to form sounds. Although esophageal speech does not result in smooth sounds, it is the first step in learning pharyngeal speech. In pharyngeal speech, the individual blocks the air that enters the nose and mouth with quick tongue actions, causing it to vibrate against the pharynx (the empty space in the throat above the larynx). Pharyngeal speech requires a great deal of patience and practice before the speech approaches the sounds of normal speech.

A *cleft palate* is a split or fissure in the roof of the mouth. Cleft palate interferes with the formation of consonants, which are formed by pressure of the tongue on the roof of the mouth. Cleft palate is usually corrected by surgery. However, even individuals who have undergone successful surgery may still have speech impairments.

Cerebral palsy, a condition in which nerve tissues in the brain are defective or injured, results in partial paralysis and lack of muscle control. There are many varieties of cerebral palsy; those that cause respiratory problems frequently result in speech impairments. Because cerebral palsy is a central nervous system disorder, the effects on speech are generally those involving the motor mechanisms of speech (Weiss and Lillywhite: 1981).

PSYCHOLOGICAL ASPECTS OF SPEECH IMPAIRMENTS

The psychological responses to speech impairments vary with the type of impairment. Parents of children who are deaf or hearing impaired or who have cerebral palsy may find it overwhelming to learn about these conditions and the services available to help their children At the same time, they must learn to cope with necessary changes in the family's way of living. Individuals who have cancer must learn to speak in a different way while they are facing the possible recurrence of the disease. Laryngectomees and individuals who stutter fear that they will be unable to communicate in everyday situations and worry about embarrassment. In addition, people who cannot speak fear that they will not be able to obtain help in case of an emergency. People with aphasia often have multiple disorders, since aphasia is usually caused by stroke or traumatic brain injury. Depression is common and natural under these circumstances. Many people assume that individuals who cannot communicate verbally also lack normal intelligence. This inaccurate stereotype leads to further loss of self-esteem for the person who is nonverbal.

The *speech-language pathologist* aids in the recovery or maintenance of speech or language function. Speech-language pathologists conduct screenings to detect possible speech impairments. After an assessment of the condition, the speech-language pathologist designs and implements a program to treat the individual's language difficulties. Often the test results obtained by the speech-language pathologist will help the medical staff in caring for the individual with aphasia. Speech-language pathologists may have sub-specialties, so it is important to find one who has experience in the specific condition. Speech-language pathologists are certified by the American Speech-Language-Hearing Association (ASHA) and receive a certificate of clinical competence (CCC).

Other service providers who work with speech-language pathologists include *audiologists,* who help to determine whether hearing impairment is a contributory factor; *special educators*, who may help the speech-language pathologists determine the appropriate educational program for children; and *otolaryngologists,* who diagnose and treat the physical conditions affecting the ears and throat. *Social workers* may help individuals with speech impairments in various ways, including locating appropriate service providers and helping individuals to overcome their fears and embarrassments. *Psychologists* provide counseling to help individuals overcome denial, accept changes that have occurred in their lives, and learn how to cope effectively. *Vocational rehabilitation counselors* help individuals find services and assistive devices to enable them to remain independent and find appropriate job placements.

WHERE TO FIND SERVICES

Both speech-language pathologists and audiologists work in schools; speech and hearing clinics; rehabilitation units at hospitals; and private practices. Many colleges and universities that train speech-language pathologists and audiologists also operate clinics where they provide services to the public. The American Speech-Language-Hearing Association (ASHA) provides a free list of certified speech-language pathologists and audiologists in each state. Public school systems generally hire both speech-language pathologists and audiologists as regular staff members to provide services to students. State supported vocational rehabilitation agencies, otolaryngology departments, and rehabilitation units at hospitals also offer these services.

ASSISTIVE DEVICES

Devices that enable people with speech impairments to communicate are referred to as augmentative communication devices. Communication boards depict symbols that represent words or ideas; people who are unable to speak may point to the symbols to communicate. Speech synthesizers (which are also used by people who are visually impaired or blind) are artificial voices that utilize modern technology; they may be built into a communication board or they may be part of a computer system. When part of a computer system, they may be used with a variety of options, such as printers, keyboards, and headpointers for people with limited mobility.

Portable communication aids operate on batteries and enable the user to locate words or phrases that are pronounced by a speech synthesizer. For people who have mobility impairments as well as speech impairments, switches are available to facilitate the use of these devices. Different types of switches are designed for operation by different parts of the body. For example, puff switches are activated by blowing into a mouthpiece; others may be operated by the hands or the feet; and still others may be mounted on wheelchairs.

Personal computers with speech synthesizers may be used in conjunction with software programs to train individuals with speech impairments to improve their verbal skills. These programs help with articulation, stuttering, pitch, and rate, and provide evaluative feedback of the individual's speech. Special programs have been developed for impairments caused by various conditions, such as aphasia and brain injury, and for children. Special instructional programs for children who have not developed speech use pictures along with communication boards that say the word associated with the picture. Some speech synthesizers connected to computers enable individuals with speech impairments to communicate over the telephone. Telecommunication devices for the deaf (TDD's) may also be used for phone communication by anyone who is unable to speak.

Portable speech amplifiers are available for people who have had laryngectomies. Devices to help people who have had laryngectomies learn to use their esophageal voice and artificial larynxes are also available.

References

Albert, Martin and Nancy Helm-Estabrooks
1988   "Diagnosis and Treatment of Aphasia, Part II" JAMA 259(Feb 26):8: 1205-1210

Bernstein, Lynne E., Moise H. Goldstein, and James J. Mahshie
1990 "Speech Training Aids for Hearing-Impaired Individuals: Overview and Aims" Journal of Rehabilitation Research 25(4):53-62

Bowe, Frank
1978 Handicapping America New York: Harper and Row

Fraser, Malcolm
1990 Self-Therapy for the Stutterer Memphis, TN: Speech Foundation of America

Kriegman, Lois
1978 "Speech and Language Disorders" pp. 541-559 in Robert M. Goldenson (ed.) <u>Disability and Rehabilitation Handbook</u> New York: McGraw Hill

Schwartz, Sue
1987 <u>Choices in Deafness: A Parents Guide</u> Kensington, MD: Woodbine House

U.S. Bureau of the Census
1986 <u>Disability, Functional Limitation, and Health Insurance Coverage: 1984/85</u> Current Population Reports, Series P-70, No. 8, Washington, DC: U.S. Government Printing Office

Weiss, Curtis E. and Herold S. Lillywhite
1981 <u>Communicative Disorders: Prevention and Early Intervention</u> St. Louis: C.V. Mosby

ORGANIZATIONS

(In the listings below, telephone numbers have symbols V for voice and TDD for tele-communication device for the deaf where organizations have published this information.)

<u>American Speech-Language-Hearing Association</u> (ASHA)
10801 Rockville Pike
Rockville, MD 20852
(800) 638-8255   (301) 897-5700 (V/TDD)

A professional organization of speech and language pathologists and audiologists. Provides information on communication problems and a free list of certified audiologists and speech therapists for each state. Toll free HELPLINE offers answers to questions about conditions and services as well as referrals.

<u>Council for Exceptional Children</u> (CEC)
1920 Association Drive
Reston, VA 22091
(703) 620-3660

A professional membership organization that works toward improving the quality of education for children who have disabilities or are gifted; special division for communication disorders. Regular membership, $55.00

<u>Courage Stroke Network</u>
3915 Golden Valley Road
Golden Valley, MN 55422
(800) 553-6321

An information network for people who have had a stroke and their families. Helps establish local stroke groups, conducts seminars for consumers and professionals, and publishes fact sheet, "Helping a Stroke Survivor Who has Aphasia Communicate;" a membership newsletter, "Stroke Connection," and a penpal newsletter for members with aphasia, "A Stroke of Luck." Membership for stroke survivors, $7.00 (courtesy membership available for those who cannot afford membership fee); professionals, $15.00

<u>Heart and Stroke Foundation of Canada</u>
160 George Street, Suite 200
Ottawa, Ontario K1N 9M2 Canada
(613) 237-4361

Conducts research and professional and public education through provincial divisions and chapters. Free publications list.

International Association of Laryngectomees
c/o American Cancer Society
1599 Clifton Road, NE
Atlanta, GA 30329
(404) 320-3333

Sponsors self-help groups throughout the United States and disseminates information through its publications. "First Steps: Helping Words for the Laryngectomee" is a booklet with information about surgery, speech therapy, and sources of equipment. Free

National Aphasia Association
400 East 34th Street, Room RR 306
New York, NY 10016

Provides information about aphasia and resources for patients and family members. Develops support groups and promotes clinical research. Individual membership, $25.00

National Center for Stuttering
200 Est 33rd Street
New York, NY 10016
(800) 221-2483   In NY, (212) 532-1460

Trains stutterers to use new technique of breathing to relax vocal cords. Provides training for speech professionals. Hotline answers questions about stuttering.

National Easter Seal Society
70 East Lake Street
Chicago, IL 60601
(312) 726-6200   (312) 726-4258 (TDD)

Promotes research, education, and rehabilitation for people with physical disabilities and speech and language problems. Sponsors Easter Seal Stroke Clubs for people who have had strokes, their families, and friends.

National Institute of Neurological Disorders and Stroke
National Institutes of Health
Information Office
Building 31, Room 8A06
9000 Rockville Pike
Bethesda, MD 20892
(301) 496-5751

A federal agency that supports basic and clinical research on brain and nervous system disorders.

National Institute on Deafness and Other Communication Disorders
National Institutes of Health
Building 31, Room 1B-62
9000 Rockville Pike
Bethesda, MD 20892
(301) 496-7243   (301) 492-0252 (TDD)

Federal agency that funds basic research studies on problems of hearing, balance, voice, language, and speech.

National Stroke Association
300 East Hampden Avenue, Suite 240
Englewood, CO 80110-2622
(303) 762-9922

Assists individuals with stroke and educates their families, physicians, and the general public about stroke. Publishes "Effective Communication with the Aphasic Person," a pamphlet with tips on communicating with individuals who are aphasic, and a quarterly newsletter, "Be Stroke Smart."

Rehabilitation Engineering Center on Augmentative Communication
Department of Computer and Information Science
University of Delaware
Newark, DE 19711
(302) 451-2712

A federally funded center that conducts research into the development of print and synthetic speech communication aids.

Rehabilitation R & D Center
VA Medical Center
3801 Miranda Avenue/ 153
Palo Alto, CA 94304-1200

Develops assistive devices, including computer systems for aphasics. Publishes, "OnCenter," a newsletter that discusses recent developments at the center, free.

Speech Foundation of America
PO Box 11749
Memphis, TN 38111-0479
(800) 992-9392

Dedicated to the prevention of stuttering in children and improved treatment for adults. Hotline answers questions about stuttering. Provides information packet and referrals for parents of children who stutter. Maintains a national list of referrals. Conducts conferences for professionals. Produces numerous publications and videotapes about stuttering.

Stroke Recovery Association
170 The Donway West, Suite 122A
Don Mills, Ontario M3C 2G3 Canada
(416) 441-1421

This organization of individuals who have had strokes and health care professionals provides information and emotional support to people who have had strokes and their families. Publishes the "Phoenix," a monthly magazine. Membership, $15.00 per family.

United Cerebral Palsy Association (UCPA)
7 Penn Plaza
New York, NY 10001
(800) 872-1827   (212) 481-6300

Member groups throughout the country provide treatment, information, education, and counseling.

After a Stroke
Resources for Rehabilitation
33 Bedford Street, Suite 19A
Lexington, MA 02173
(617) 862-6455

Designed for distribution by professionals to people with disabilities, this publication includes information on how to obtain services, organizations that serve people who have had strokes, publications, and assistive devices. Minimum purchase 25 copies. $2.00 per copy. See order form opposite inside back cover.

Children with Speech and Language Difficulties
by Alec Webster and Christine McConnell
Brookes Publishing Company
PO Box 10624
Baltimore, MD 21285-9945
(800) 638-3775

This book develops a conceptual model of speech and language development and provides information about assessment materials. $21.50

Developmental Speech and Language Disorders: Hope through Research
National Institute on Deafness and Other Communication Disorders
National Institutes of Health
Building 31, Room 1B-62
9000 Rockville Pike
Bethesda, MD 20892
(301) 496-7243   (301) 492-0252 (TDD)

Booklet describing the types and causes of speech disorders, treatment, and research. Free

If Your Child Stutters
Speech Foundation of America
PO Box 11749
Memphis, TN 38111-0479
(800) 992-9392

A guide that enables parents to provide appropriate help for children who stutter. $1.00

Journal of Rehabilitation Research and Development (JRRD)
Office of Technology Transfer
VA Prosthetics R&D Center
103 South Gay Street
Baltimore, MD 21202

A quarterly publication of scientific and engineering articles including those related to augmentative communication devices. Includes abstracts of literature, book reviews, and calendar of events. For sale by U.S. Superintendent of Documents, Government Printing Office, Washington DC 20402

Parents' Guide to Speech and Deafness
by Donald R. Calvert
Alexander Graham Bell Association for the Deaf
3417 Volta Place, NW
Washington, DC 20007-2778
(202) 337-5220 (V/TDD)

A guide to help parents play an active role in the speech development of children with hearing impairment. $9.50 plus $2.00 shipping and handling

Self-Therapy for the Stutterer
by Malcolm Fraser
Speech Foundation of America
PO Box 11749
Memphis, TN 38111-0479
(800) 992-9392

A guide to help adults who stutter overcome the problems on their own. $3.00

Stuttering: Hope through Research
National Institute on Deafness and Other Communication Disorders
National Institutes of Health
Building 31, Room 1B-62
9000 Rockville Pike
Bethesda, MD 20892
(301) 496-7243   (301) 492-0252 (TDD)

Describes how speech is produced, treatments for stuttering, and research supported by the federal government.

(In the listings below, telephone numbers have symbols V for voice and TDD for tele-communication device for the deaf where organizations have published this information.)

Communication Aids for Children and Adults
Crestwood Company
6625 North Sidney Place
Milwaukee WI 53209
(414) 352-5678

Mail order catalogue with a wide variety of teaching aids for children and adults with speech impairments, toys, switches, and other products for people who have both speech and mobility impairments. Free

Communication Skill Builders
3830 East Bellevue, PO Box 42050-E91
Tucson, AZ 85733
(602) 323-7500

Mail order catalogue with a wide variety of products for children and adults with speech impairments and evaluative tools for professionals. Free

Don Johnston Developmental Equipment
PO Box 639
1000 North Rand Road, Building 115
Wauconda, IL 60084-0639
(800) 999-4660   (708) 526-2682

Mail order catalogue of communication boards, speech synthesizers used in conjunction with software programs that teach speech, adapted computer equipment, and publications. Free

Imaginart Communication Products
307 Arizona Street
Bisbee, AZ 85603
(800) 828-1376   (602) 432-5741

Mail order catalogue of augmentative communication devices for children and adults; special products for people with traumatic brain injury, aphasia, and cleft palate; videotapes; and books. Free

Jesana Ltd.
PO Box 17
Irvington, NY 10533
(800) 443-4728

Mail order catalogue of speech aids, language software, adapted toys and devices, and other products for children with disabilities.

Prentke Romich
1022 Heyl Road
Wooster, OH 44691
(800) 262-1984   (216) 262-1984

Produces augmentative communication systems and alternative computer access devices. Provides training in the use of their products.

Resource Guide for Persons with Speech or Language Impairments
IBM National Support Center for Persons with Disabilities
PO Box 2150
Atlanta, GA 30301-2150
(800) 426-2133 (V)   (800) 284-9482 (TDD)

Describes products used with IBM personal computers, including software programs to train people to improve their speech and stand alone communication devices. Free

STANTON ADD*vox*™ II

A Personal Amplifier/Speaker System for Speech Enhancement and Voice Projection

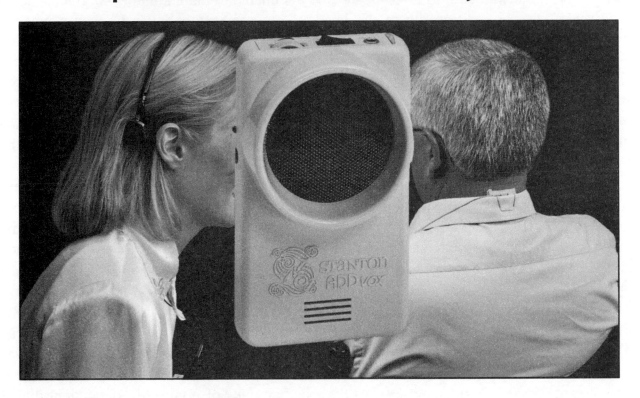

The Stanton **ADD***vox*™ II amplifier/speaker system is an improved body worn amplifier/speaker intended for use with the Stanton M.I.T. (Miniature Inertial Transducer).

The primary application is for speech enhancement of those who have difficulty projecting their voice, and where a microphone in front of the lips is impractical.

The system consists of an amplifier speaker box with bandpass filters and A.V.C. It also contains a separate on/off switch and adjustable volume control. The M.I.T. is mounted in a neckband or in a headband assembly. An accessory extension cable, a neck lanyard, four Ni-Cad batteries and a recharger adaptor are included.

For pricing information and purchasing procedures, contact:

Personal Communications Division,

STANTON MAGNETICS

101 Sunnyside Boulevard, Plainview, NY 11803
Phone 516/349-0235   Fax 516/349-0230

Toll Free 1-800-526-3684

DIABETES

Diabetes mellitus is a term that applies to a variety of disorders where the insulin mechanism is abnormal and, as a result, the body is unable to maintain normal glucose levels. *Hypoglycemia* is a condition where the level of glucose is too low. It occurs when the individual does not eat soon enough or eats too little, uses too much insulin, or engages in overactivity. Hypoglycemia may lead to an insulin reaction; symptoms may include feeling shaky or sweaty, headache, hunger, irritability, and dizziness. Insulin shock sometimes occurs if an insulin reaction is not treated quickly; in these cases individuals may lose consciousness. *Hyperglycemia* is a condition where the level of glucose in the blood is too high. Symptoms include extreme thirst, a dry mouth, excessive urination, blurred vision, and lethargy. Sometimes when an individual who has had an insulin reaction takes food high in sugar to replace glucose in the body, too much glucose is released, resulting in high blood sugar levels (hyperglycemia). The combination of too much sugar without enough insulin to use it properly may gradually lead to diabetic coma if warning signs are not monitored. Hyperglycemia is less common than hypoglycemia, and diabetic coma usually occurs only in insulin-dependent diabetes.

According to self-reports, there are nearly seven million cases of known diabetes in the United States (Centers for Disease Control: 1990). The prevalence rate is 24.7 cases of diabetes per thousand for the entire population (National Center for Health Statistics: 1986). It is estimated that half of the Americans age 65 or older who have diabetes are not aware of it (Friedman: 1986). African-Americans have higher rates of noninsulin-dependent diabetes mellitus (NIDDM) than white non-Hispanic Americans, and diabetes is now the third leading cause of death by disease for African-Americans (National Institute of Diabetes and Digestive and Kidney Diseases: 1990).

Diabetes and its complications are responsible for many hospital stays and have a large economic impact on society. Although there is no cure for diabetes, there are means to control the disease and to decrease the risk of the numerous associated complications. Early diagnosis and intervention are crucial steps in maintaining proper control of diabetes.

TYPES OF DIABETES

The two major types of diabetes mellitus are referred to as Type I and Type II. In *Type I*, the pancreas does not produce insulin, a substance that is necessary to metabolize the glucose (sugar) that the body needs for energy. Individuals with Type I diabetes must take regular injections of insulin. For this reason, Type I is also referred to as Insulin-Dependent Diabetes Mellitus (IDDM). This variant of the disease was formerly called juvenile-onset diabetes, because it is usually diagnosed at a young age.

In the United States there are an estimated 300,000 to 500,00 individuals with Insulin-Dependent Diabetes Mellitus (National Institute of Diabetes and Digestive and Kidney Diseases: 1990). In addition to daily insulin injections, individuals with IDDM must carefully watch their diet and coordinate meals with insulin doses to maintain a balanced glucose level. Many people use home blood glucose monitoring equipment to measure glucose levels. Long-term complications of IDDM include kidney, heart, and eye disease, as well as nerve damage (diabetic neuropathy).

In *Type II* diabetes, the body produces some insulin but does not produce enough or does not utilize it properly. Because Type II diabetes does not require insulin injections, it is also referred to as noninsulin-dependent diabetes mellitus (NIDDM). This type of the disease is often called adult-onset or maturity-onset diabetes, because most frequently it is diagnosed after age forty. It is estimated that over 90% of the cases of diabetes in the United States are Type II (NCHS: 1987).

Although the causes of Type II diabetes are not known, obesity and a family history of diabetes are predisposing factors. Symptoms of noninsulin-dependent diabetes include fatigue, frequent urination, and excessive thirst. Individuals who have these symptoms should make an appointment for a physical examination. It should be pointed out, however, that diabetes is sometimes present when no symptoms are evident (Williams: 1983). In many cases, noninsulin-dependent diabetes can be controlled through both diet and exercise.

Diet and exercise for people with either type of diabetes should be planned with a physician's advice to insure that all medical conditions are taken into account. The goals of dietary restrictions are to reduce total body weight and to minimize the intake of glucose. The American Diabetes Association has produced many publications about diet for people with diabetes, including "Exchange Lists," which list foods with similar caloric and nutrient contents (See "PUBLICATIONS AND TAPES" section below). Exercise helps the body to burn off the glucose and thus is an important part of the plan to control diabetes. After consulting with a physician, even individuals who have been sedentary can begin a gradual exercise program by starting to take brief daily walks.

People with diabetes monitor their blood glucose by putting a drop of blood on a specially treated paper strip designed to react to the glucose. The color of the strip indicates the level of glucose that is present. Color charts that indicate colors of high, normal, and low glucose are used for comparison with the strips. Machines with LED displays or speech output, called glucometers, are also available to read the strips.

Both types of diabetes have the same potential long-term health effects. It is essential that everyone with diabetes be aware of the proper management of their disease and all of the potential complications. Complications of diabetes include greater risks of heart disease, stroke, infections, and kidney disease; circulatory problems that can be especially problematic for legs and feet (resulting in amputation in extreme cases); neuropathy or nerve disease which causes tingling, numbness, double vision, pain, or dizziness; and vision problems.

Among the leading vision problems caused by diabetes is diabetic retinopathy. Visual impairment occurs when the small blood vessels in the retina are damaged and fail to nourish the retina adequately. One consequence of this process is bleeding inside the eye. If detected early, diabetic retinopathy can sometimes be treated successfully by laser therapy. In other cases, complex surgical procedures are performed in the attempt to restore useful vision. To manage their diabetes, many people with visual impairments use a wide range of adapted equipment such as "talking" glucometers, scales, and thermometers; syringe magnifiers, special insulin gauges, and special syringes that automatically measure insulin doses.

DIABETES IN CHILDREN

In youth under the age of 17, the rate of known diabetes is .9 per thousand (National Center for Health Statistics: 1986). Childhood diabetes (Type I or IDDM) is often first diagnosed by a family physician, usually after an acute episode marked by extreme thirst, unexplained weight loss, and/or frequent urination. Children with diabetes are often referred to a pediatric diabetes specialist or to a specialty clinic for training in the management of their condition.

Children with diabetes should be taught to accept the major responsibility for control of their disease. School personnel should be informed about the student's diabetes and should know the warning signs of an insulin reaction and what measures to take if an insulin reaction occurs. Generally there is no need to avoid participation in sports; however, extra carbohydrates may be needed after strenuous activity.

Children with diabetes often attend a "diabetes" camp where they can meet other children with diabetes. In such a setting, children can learn how to cope effectively and discuss their feelings about diabetes. Attendance at a camp for children with diabetes also provides the family with a respite period. Family support groups also offer valuable practical information and emotional support. Other children in the family may feel neglected when parents are concentrating on the care of a sibling with diabetes.

DIABETES IN ELDERS

The prevalence of NIDDM for persons 65 years and older is 88.4 per thousand (National Center for Health Statistics: 1986). A quarter of African-American adults age 65 to 74 has diabetes. As might be expected, the rate of severe complications is also higher; amputations, visual impairment, and kidney disease are more prevalent in African-Americans than in whites (National Institute of Diabetes and Digestive and Kidney Disease: 1990).

Elders, especially those who live alone, must understand the importance of their diet in diabetes control. If they receive meals-on-wheels or attend a senior meal site, they should make known their special dietary needs. Senior health programs which include screenings for hypertension, diabetes, and vision problems; foot care programs; and exercise classes may help reduce the incidence of diabetes complications. (For a more detailed description of diabetes in elders, see Resources for Elders with Disabilities, described in "PUBLICATIONS AND TAPES" section below.)

PSYCHOLOGICAL ASPECTS OF DIABETES

Although shock, fear, and depression are normal reactions to diabetes at first, these emotions may subside once the individual understands how to control the disease. Many people feel a loss of control over their bodies. Because diabetes affects so many parts of the body, it also affects many aspects of daily life. In addition to prescribed changes in diet and exercise, individuals with diabetes must always be aware of the symptoms that indicate hyperglycemia or hypoglycemia.

Changes in daily routines are never accepted readily. For individuals with diabetes, changes in lifestyle and the need to monitor glucose may cause great stress. Social events and travel must be carefully planned to insure that meals will comply with special diets. Glucose monitoring equipment must be packed for travel and arrangements made to carry out regular monitoring activities.

The child with Type I diabetes usually adjusts quickly to insulin injections, and even young children learn to administer their own insulin. Adolescents with diabetes may worry about being different from their peers at a time of life when conformity is highly valued. It is common for all adolescents to worry about school, social life, and the future; for adolescents with diabetes, an additional variable makes the stress greater. Illness, even a simple cold, can affect how the body uses insulin; glucose monitoring is even more important at these times.

Parents of children with Type I diabetes must cope with the knowledge that their child has a chronic disease; they may have the same feelings as an adult who has just been diagnosed as having diabetes. Although the exact cause of diabetes is still unknown, parents often feel guilty that their child may have inherited traits that put him or her at risk for diabetes. Families must adjust to the strict schedule of meals, injections, and monitoring necessary to manage their child's diabetes. Parents must try not to be over-protective and should allow their children to participate in normal recreational activities.

Diligent efforts to control glucose by following the recommended dosages of insulin do not always result in the desired response. Individuals whose glucose is out of control should learn not to feel guilty; they may need to have their dosage and diet modified by a health care professional.

A common response to adult-onset or Type II diabetes is that "It's just a touch of diabetes." This response can be extremely dangerous when the individual fails to properly monitor and control the disease. Individuals with diabetes and their family members must discuss the disease and its potential effects so that they understand the importance of the prescribed dietary regimen, exercise, and blood glucose monitoring. It should not be assumed that children or elders with diabetes are not capable of caring for themselves properly solely because of their age. Family members should be instructed to allow these individuals to have the maximum responsibility possible for caring for themselves. Although individuals should understand their own responsibility for following the prescribed regimen to control diabetes, they should not be made to feel guilty when their glucose is out of control.

PROFESSIONAL SERVICE PROVIDERS

Because diabetes is a systemic disease, it has a wide range of effects. As a result, many types of health care professionals are involved in caring for people with diabetes.

Diabetologists (endocrinologists) are physicians who specialize in the treatment of individuals with diabetes and coordinate the various aspects of care for patients with diabetes. *Nephrologists* are physicians who treat people with kidney disease, which is a common complication of diabetes. *Ophthalmologists* are physicians who specialize in diseases of the eye. If diabetic retinopathy is detected, individuals are often referred to subspecialists called retina and vitreous specialists.

Certified Diabetes Educators (CDE) are health care professionals certified by the American Association of Diabetes Educators to teach individuals with diabetes how to effectively manage their disease. Certified diabetes educators may be physicians or nurses. Many are dieticians or nutritionists who help people with diabetes plan a diet to control their blood glucose levels.

Psychologists, *social workers*, and other counselors help people with diabetes and their family members adjust to the regimen prescribed to control the diabetes.

WHERE TO FIND SERVICES

In some areas, special treatment centers for diabetes and dialysis centers for people with kidney disease are available. The special physicians listed above practice in hospitals or have private practices. Affiliates of the American Diabetes Association (ADA) exist in every state. These affiliates may provide publications, educational programs, sponsor camps for children with diabetes, and make referrals to local resources. The national office (described in "ORGANIZATIONS" section below) can provide the address and phone number of local affiliates. The ADA also has information about support groups that individuals can join. Understanding that others with diabetes continue to live fulfilling lives can be an extremely

110

important benefit of attending support groups. People with diabetes who have vision problems may obtain services from public or private rehabilitation agencies serving individuals who are visually impaired or blind (see Chapter 11, "Visual Impairment and Blindness").

ASSISTIVE DEVICES

Individuals with insulin-dependent diabetes use a variety of devices to administer their insulin, such as syringes; insulin pens which combine the insulin dose and injector; needle-free jet injectors; and insulin pumps, which deliver insulin slowly throughout the day and night through a plastic tube attached to a needle. Equipment to measure sugar in urine and blood glucose monitors are necessary for both Type I and Type II forms of diabetes. These are usually prescribed by medical professionals, so this chapter will not go into detail about these devices. Some health insurance policies will pay some of the costs for glucose meters and test strips. Check with your insurance carrier before purchasing such equipment.

HOW TO RECOGNIZE AN INSULIN REACTION AND GIVE FIRST AID

Individuals experiencing an insulin reaction may feel shaky or dizzy, sweat profusely, complain of a headache, or act irritable. Suggestions for giving first aid to individuals who have had an insulin reaction are:

- Give the individual some food, such as orange juice, milk, or even sugar itself, to replace the low blood sugar level. Many individuals with diabetes carry sugar packets or candy with them for use in emergencies.

- If the individual is unconscious, rub honey or another sugary substance into the mouth, between the teeth and cheek.

- After an insulin reaction, the individual should eat a piece of fruit, sandwich, or other snack to prevent the high level of insulin created by emergency treatment from causing another reaction.

Frequent insulin reactions should be reported to the physician. It is recommended that individuals with diabetes wear a medical identification bracelet so that emergency care personnel will know that they have diabetes.

References

Centers for Disease Control
1990 <u>Diabetes Surveillance, 1980-1987</u> Atlanta, GA: Centers for Disease Control

Friedman, JoAnn
1986 <u>Home Health Care</u> New York: W. W. Norton

Juvenile Diabetes Foundation International
no   "Information About Insulin" New York: Juvenile Diabetes Foundation International
date

National Center for Health Statistics
1987 "Health Practices and Perceptions of U.S. Adults with Noninsulin-Dependent Diabetes.
       Data from the 1985 National Health Interview Survey of Health Promotion and Disease
       Prevention" <u>Advance Data from Vital and Health Statistics</u>, No. 141, DHHS Pub. No.
       (PHS) 87-1250. Public Health Service, Hyattsville, MD September 23, 1987
1986 "Prevalence, Impact, and Demography of Known Diabetes in the United States"
       <u>Advance Data from Vital and Health Statistics</u>, No. 114, DHHS Pub. No. (PHS) 86-
       1250. Public Health Service, Hyattsville, MD February 12, 1986

National Institute of Diabetes and Digestive and Kidney Diseases
1990a <u>Diabetes-Related Programs for Black Americans: A Resource Guide</u> NIH Publication
       No. 90-1585. Bethesda, MD: National Diabetes Information Clearinghouse
1990b "Insulin-Dependent Diabetes" Bethesda, MD: National Diabetes Information Clear-
       inghouse

Williams, T. Franklin
1983 "Diabetes Mellitus in Older People" pp. 411-415 in William Reichel (ed.) <u>Clinical
       Aspects of Aging</u> Baltimore, MD: Williams and Wilkins

ORGANIZATIONS

(In the listings below, telephone numbers have symbols V for voice and TDD for tele-communication device for the deaf where organizations have published this information.)

American Diabetes Association (ADA)
1660 Duke Street
Alexandria, VA 22314
(800) 232-3472   In Washington DC, (703) 549-1500

National membership organization with local affiliates. Publications for both professionals and individuals, including cookbooks and guides for the management of diabetes (See "PUBLIC-ATIONS AND TAPES" section below). $24.00 annual membership fee includes discounts on many publications, and subscription to "Diabetes Forecast" (Also available on disc from the National Library Service. See Chapter 11, "Visual Impairment and Blindness"). Many local affiliates offer their own publications, sponsor support groups, and conduct professional train-ing programs.

Canadian Diabetes Association
78 Bond Street
Toronto, Ontario M5B 2J8 Canada
(416) 362-4440

Provides service and education to individuals with diabetes; serves as an advocate, and provides support for research.

Juvenile Diabetes Foundation International (JDF)
The Diabetes Research Foundation
432 Park Avenue South
New York, NY 10016-8013
(800) 533-2873   (212) 889-7575

Supports research and provides information to individuals with diabetes and their families. Chapters in many states and affiliates in other countries. Annual membership, $25.00, includes quarterly magazine, "Countdown."

National Diabetes Information Clearinghouse (NDIC)
Box NDIC
Bethesda, MD 20892
(301) 468-2162

Responds to information requests from the public and professionals. Maintains a database of publications and brochures. Publishes bimonthly newsletter, "Diabetes Dateline," free. Free list of publications (See "PUBLICATIONS AND TAPES" section below).

National Institute of Diabetes and Digestive and Kidney Diseases
National Institutes of Health
Bethesda, MD 20892

Funds basic and clinical research in the causes, prevention, and treatment of diabetes. Free list of publications.

<u>Audiovisual Resources for Diabetes</u>
Learning Resource Center
University of Michigan Medical School
1135 East Catherine Street
Ann Arbor, MI 48109-0726
(313) 763-6770

Annotated catalogue of audiovisual materials. $30.00 prepaid; $35.00 with a purchase order.

<u>Buyer's Guide to Diabetes Products</u>
American Diabetes Association (ADA)
1970 Chain Bridge Road
McLean, VA 22109-0592
(800) 232-3472   In Washington DC area, (703) 549-1500

Comparison of prices and features for a wide variety of products for people with diabetes.
Members, $1.80; nonmembers, $2.00 plus $1.75 shipping and handling.

<u>Children with Diabetes</u>
by Linda M. Siminerio and Jean Betschart
American Diabetes Association
1970 Chain Bridge Road
McLean, VA 22109-0592
(800) 232-3472   In Washington DC area, (703) 549-1500

Written for children with diabetes and their families, this book offers a special perspective on diabetes in youth. Members, $7.15; nonmembers, $7.95; plus $3.00 shipping and handling.

"Diabetes and Vision Loss: Special Considerations"
by Marla Bernbaum, MD
<u>Providing Services for People with Vision Loss, Volume 2</u>
Resources for Rehabilitation
33 Bedford Street, Suite 19A
Lexington, MA 02173
(617) 862-6455

Provides information on the psychosocial implications and special rehabilitation needs of individuals with vision loss due to diabetes. $24.95 plus $3.00 shipping and handling.

<u>Diabetes: Caring for Your Emotions As Well as Your Health</u>
by Jerry Edelwich and Archie Brodsky
Addison Wesley Publishing Company, Reading, MA

This book offers suggestions for adaptation, relationships with medical personnel, family strategies, employment questions, technology, and support groups. $12.95

Diabetes Self-Management
150 West 22nd Street
New York, NY 10011

A bimonthly magazine to help people with diabetes manage their disease. Tips on diet, foot care, medical news, etc. $18.00

The Diabetes Sourcebook
by Diana W. Guthrie and Richard A. Guthrie
Lowell House
1875 Century Park East, Suite 220
Los Angeles, CA 90067

Describes diabetes, its complications, psychological issues, and suggestions for the individuals' management of their disease. Includes a list of camps for children with diabetes. $21.95

Diabetes Teaching Guide for People Who Use Insulin
Joslin Diabetes Center
One Joslin Place
Boston, MA 02215

Discusses the causes of diabetes, the role of diet and exercise, meal planning, and complications. Also provides information on drawing, mixing, and injecting insulin. $20.00

Diabetes Treatment with Insulin: A Short Guide
Diabetes Treatment without Insulin: A Short Guide
Joslin Diabetes Center
One Joslin Place
Boston, MA 02215

Written for individuals with diabetes who read at a fourth grade level or those who speak English as a second language. Each publication, $8.50

Diabetes Type II: Living a Long, Healthy Life through Blood-Sugar Normalization
by Richard K. Bernstein
Prentice Hall Press, New York, NY

Written by a physician who has diabetes himself, this book discusses control of blood sugar, diet, medication, and exercise. $18.45

The Diabetic Dictionary
National Diabetes Information Clearinghouse (NDIC)
Box NDIC
Bethesda, MD 20892
(301) 468-2162

A glossary of terms diabetics are likely to encounter; written in simple language. Single copy, free.

Diabetic Retinopathy
National Eye Institute (NEI)
Building 31, Room 6A32
Bethesda, MD 20892
(301) 496-5248

Discusses the effects of diabetes on the eyes: symptoms, treatment, and vitrectomy. Free. Also available in large print (free) or on cassette ($2.00) from VISION Foundation, Inc., 818 Mt. Auburn Street, Watertown, MA 02172

The Diabetic Traveler
PO Box 8223 RW
Stamford, CT 06905
(203) 327-5832

Quarterly newsletter for individuals with diabetes, $15.00. Sample issue $1.00, with a self-addressed stamped envelope.

Diabetic's Book: All Your Questions Answered
by June Bierman and Barbara Toohey
St Martin's Press, New York, NY

Discusses a wide variety of issues affecting people with diabetes, including diet, exercise, emotions, and other aspects of everyday living. $10.95

Exchange Lists for Meal Planning
American Diabetes Association
1970 Chain Bridge Road
McLean, VA 22109-0592
(800) 232-3472   In Washington DC area, (703) 549-1500

These guidelines for nutrition and meal planning list foods that are similar in caloric and nutrient content. Standard print, $1.30, plus $1.75 shipping and handling; large print, $2.50, plus $1.75 shipping and handling.

Grilled Cheese at Four O'Clock in the Morning
by Judy Miller
American Diabetes Association (ADA)
1970 Chain Bridge Road
McLean, VA 22109-0592
(800) 232-3472   In Washington DC area, (703) 549-1500

Written for children with diabetes and their families, this publication discusses diabetes in youth. Members, $5.35; nonmembers, $5.95; plus $3.00 shipping and handling.

If Your Child Has Diabetes: An Answer Book for Parents
by Joanne Elliott
Putnam Publishing Group
200 Madison Avenue
New York, NY 10016

Provides information and recommendations for parents of children with diabetes on subjects such as school, recreation, medical and life insurance, and employment as well as general information about diabetes. U.S., $9.95; Canada, $12.95

Insulin-Dependent Diabetes
National Diabetes Information Clearinghouse (NDIC)
Box NDIC
Bethesda, MD 20892
(301) 468-2162

A booklet written in simple language describing the prevalence, causes, long-term complications, and treatments for insulin-dependent diabetes. Single copy, free.

Know Your Diabetes, Know Yourself
Joslin Diabetes Center
One Joslin Place
Boston, MA 02215

An hour-long videotape in which Joslin patients talk about the daily issues of diabetes management - meal planning, exercise, monitoring, injections, foot and eye care, and managing the disease when sick or traveling. Joslin physicians, nurses, and other health professionals discuss the essentials of good diabetes care. VHS format. $39.95

Living with Diabetes $2.00 per copy
Living with Diabetic Retinopathy $1.75 per copy
Resources for Rehabilitation
33 Bedford Street, Suite 19A
Lexington, MA 02173
(617) 862-6455

Designed for distribution by professionals to people with diabetes, these large print (18 point bold type) publications describe the condition, service providers, organizations, devices, and publications. Minimum purchase 25 copies. See order form opposite inside back cover.

Living with Low Vision
Resources for Rehabilitation
33 Bedford Street, Suite 19A
Lexington, MA 02173
(617) 862-6455

A large print (18 point bold type) comprehensive directory that helps people with sight loss locate the services that they need to remain independent. Chapters with products that enable people to keep reading, working, and carrying out their daily activities. $35.00, plus $5.00 shipping and handling.

Managing Type II Diabetes: Your Invitation to a Healthier Lifestyle
Diabetes Center, Inc.
PO Box 739
Wayzata, MN 55391
(800) 848-2793   In Minnesota, (612) 541-0239, collect

This book addresses all aspects of diabetes management for people with noninsulin-dependent diabetes. $9.95 plus $1.50 shipping

Noninsulin-Dependent Diabetes
National Diabetes Information Clearinghouse (NDIC)
Box NDIC
Bethesda, MD 20892
(301) 468-2162

A booklet written in simple language describing the prevalence, causes, and treatments for noninsulin-dependent diabetes. Single copy, free.

Periodontal Disease and Diabetes
National Institute of Dental Research
National Institutes of Health
Bethesda, MD 20892

A brochure describing the nature of periodontal disease, its relation to diabetes, and proper care of teeth and gums for diabetics. Free

The Prevention and Treatment of Five Complications of Diabetes
National Diabetes Information Clearinghouse (NDIC)
Box NDIC
Bethesda, MD 20892
(301) 468-2162

This booklet provides an overview of the major complications and management of diabetes. $2.00

Rehabilitation Resource Manual: VISION
Resources for Rehabilitation
33 Bedford Street, Suite 19A
Lexington, MA 02173
(617) 862-6455

A desk reference that enables professionals to make effective referrals. Includes chapters on breaking the news of irreversible vision loss; guidelines on starting self-help groups; information on research and professional organizations; plus chapters on services and products for special population groups and by eye conditions and diseases. $39.95 plus $5.00 shipping and handling.

Resources for Elders with Disabilities
Resources for Rehabilitation
33 Bedford Street, Suite 19A
Lexington, MA 02173
(617) 862-6455

Provides information about services and products that older individuals with disabilities and chronic conditions need to function independently. Includes chapters on diabetes, vision loss, hearing loss, stroke, arthritis, and osteoporosis. Large print. $39.95 plus $5.00 shipping and handling.

Self Blood Glucose Monitoring
Juvenile Diabetes Foundation International
432 Park Avenue South
New York, NY 10016
(800) 223-1138   (212) 889-7575

A brochure describing the process and benefits of self blood glucose monitoring. Free

<u>The Voice of the Diabetic</u>
National Federation of the Blind (NFB)
811 Cherry Street, Suite 306
Columbia, MO 65201

A quarterly newsletter with many articles and advertisements for products used by people who have both diabetes and vision loss. Free with membership in Diabetics Division of NFB, $5.00; professional or institutional subscription, one year, $15.00; two years $28.00; three years, $40.00

EPILEPSY

Epilepsy is a condition in which the brain's cells undergo abnormal electrical activity, causing disturbances in the nervous system. An epileptic seizure occurs when there is an excessive discharge of electrical impulses from these nerve cells. Epilepsy is not a single disease or condition, nor is it contagious. It often develops in people whose families have no history of epilepsy, although children of individuals with epilepsy are thought to have a greater chance of developing this condition (Epilepsy Foundation of America: 1989).

It is estimated that 2.25 million Americans have active epilepsy, defined as seizures that are difficult to control and that require specialized care (Gumnit: 1990). About a third of the 125,000 new cases diagnosed each year occur in individuals under the age of 18 (Hauser and Hesdorffer: 1990). Individuals with severe head trauma, stroke, and infections in the central nervous system are at the greatest risk for epilepsy. Nearly half (47%) of all individuals with epilepsy have activity limitations (National Center on Health Statistics: 1988).

Physicians must have accurate information about the patient's history in order to diagnose the type of epileptic seizures and epileptic syndromes. Patients are often asked to come to the physician's office with a family member or other individual who has witnessed their seizures. Patients, family members, or friends should provide the physician with a detailed description of the seizure activity; including onset; frequency; changes in the seizures, if any; duration; and medication usage.

The electroencephalograph (EEG) is used to determine where in the brain the seizure activity is taking place. Interpretation of the EEG may help the physician determine whether the individual has epilepsy. Sometimes the EEG does not pick up the brain's electrical changes, or the patient may not have experienced any seizure activity while being monitored. In some instances, a patient may be hospitalized so that a 24 hour EEG recording may be made.

Blood tests and tests of spinal fluid are conducted to determine if an infection has caused the seizure. Tests for lead poisoning and kidney or liver disease, as well as computerized tomography scans (CT's) or magnetic resonance imaging (MRI's) may be performed to detect the presence of tumors, scar tissue, or blood clots.

TYPES OF SEIZURES

Generalized seizures affect both hemispheres of the brain and may lead to loss of consciousness, convulsions, and loss of memory. Two types of generalized seizures are the tonic-clonic and absence seizures.

A *tonic-clonic seizure* (previously called a grand mal seizure) is a generalized seizure with loss of consciousness. The individual may cry out, fall, and lie rigid. The body may jerk; bladder and bowel control may be lost; the individual may bite his or her tongue; and saliva may appear around the mouth. When the individual regains consciousness, he or she may feel sore or stiff and sleepy. The individual may or may not have any warning of the impending episode.

An *absence seizure* (previously called a petit mal seizure) is characterized by sudden onset and a blank stare. These seizures last a short time but may occur many times a day, beginning and ending abruptly. The individual is unaware of his or her surroundings and may not respond when spoken to. Sometimes speaking to the individual will stop the absence seizure.

If only one hemisphere of the brain is affected, the seizure is called a *partial seizure*. Symptoms of a partial seizure include an involuntary turning of the head, loss of speech, sweating, pallor, dilation of the pupils, and light flashes. Tingling or numbness in the face or fingers or hearing buzzing noises may also be experienced. Individuals do not lose consciousness during a partial seizure.

Complex partial seizures, which sometimes affect the temporal lobes (at the side of the brain near the ears), can also occur in several other areas of the brain. An individual having a complex partial seizure appears to be in a trance accompanied by involuntary motor activities, called *automatisms*. The individual has no control over these movements, which may include lip and tongue smacking, mimicry, hand movements, or repetitive utterances. Consciousness may or may not be impaired.

The individual is conscious during a *simple partial seizure* but cannot control body movements. An arm or leg may jerk or tremble. Seizure activity occurs in the part of the brain which controls vision, hearing, sensation, or memory. The individual may feel disoriented, fearful, or experience odd sensations on one side of the body.

An *aura* is an unusual feeling experienced by many people with epilepsy prior to a seizure. The individual may feel sick or apprehensive, have aural or visual hallucinations, or notice a peculiar odor or taste. The individual retains memory of the sensation even if he or she loses consciousness. The aura often serves as a warning that a seizure is about to take place, allowing the individual to move away from potential hazards before the onset of a major seizure.

123

TREATMENT OF EPILEPSY

Most individuals with epilepsy use *anticonvulsant or antiepileptic medications* to control seizures. The choice of antiepileptic drug is determined by the type of seizure, other clinical aspects of the seizure, the drug's side effects, cost, and method of administration. Smith (1990) recommends that drug therapy begin with a single antiepileptic drug, although the individual experiencing more than one type of seizure may need more than one drug to gain control of the seizures.

Blood level tests are used to monitor the efficacy of the chosen drug. It is important for individuals with epilepsy to maintain a fixed schedule for taking medication. Missing a dose, ceasing to take medication, or taking the wrong dosage may lead to seizure activity. Individuals taking antiepileptic medication should tell physicians treating them for other conditions about their epilepsy medicine and inquire about interactions with over-the-counter products and prescriptions.

Side effects of antiepileptic drugs may include nausea, fatigue, slurring of words, staggering, or allergic reactions (a rash or hives). Some people experience emotional changes, while others may note memory, learning, or behavior problems. Individuals should ask the physician about each drug's side effects and what to do if a reaction occurs.

Women with epilepsy who plan to become pregnant should discuss their medication with their physician, since some antiepileptic drugs have been implicated in an increase in birth defects (Epilepsy Foundation of America: 1986). Individuals should be carefully monitored during pregnancy and may expect to require some adjustment in antiepileptic medication. At least 90% of women with epilepsy who are treated with antiepileptic drugs deliver infants with no birth defects (Epilepsy Foundation of America: 1990).

Surgery may be considered when the patient's seizures always originate in one part of the brain; if medication has been unsuccessful; or when surgery will not affect vision, speech, movement, or memory. Tyler (1990) believes that surgery is not considered as often as it should be because the danger of such surgery is overestimated and the benefits underestimated. In addition, family physicians sometimes lack knowledge of specialized epilepsy surgery centers. The National Institute of Neurological Disorders and Stroke (1988) reports that more than 100,000 patients with partial seizures who do not respond to medical therapy are candidates for surgery.

A *ketogenic diet*, which is high in fat and calories, may prevent seizures in children who experience multiple side effects from standard medication. Injections of artificial adrenocorticotropic hormone (ACTH)), a substance produced by the brain to regulate the adrenal gland, may be used to manage seizures. Experimental drugs are available through special testing programs at medical epilepsy centers. The Epilepsy Foundation of America will direct individuals to a local center (see "ORGANIZATIONS" section below).

EPILEPSY IN CHILDREN

Although the frequency of newly diagnosed epilepsy in children has decreased, there are about 300,000 cases of active epilepsy in school-age children worldwide (Hauser and Hesdorffer: 1990). It is often difficult to determine the cause of seizures in children. The developmental stage of the brain, age of onset, and metabolic or genetic disorders all may influence the type of seizure.

Seizures are generally well controlled during youth, allowing medications to be withdrawn by early to middle age (Troupin and Johannessen: 1990). Epilepsy may actually disappear in some children who have experienced absence seizures only. Seizure frequency seems to decrease with age unless there is a change in the underlying cause, such as tuberous sclerosis or a brain tumor (Epilepsy Foundation of America: 1989). Currently, it is not possible to predict the course of epilepsy in any one individual.

Unfortunately, children with epilepsy rarely receive adequate information about their condition. Physicians often discuss the child's diagnosis and treatment with the parents when the child is not present. Withholding information from children may be attributed to a belief that children will not understand; that they should be protected; or that parents, rather than physicians should inform their children about their condition (Schneider and Conrad: 1983). Masland (1985) reports that overprotection, overcompensation, and rejection are common reactions of parents to children with epilepsy. He believes that the attitude of the parents plays a major role in shaping the self-image of the child who develops epilepsy. He emphasizes that the physician must provide a thorough explanation of epilepsy and its ramifications to both parent and child. Patient and family education helps children, teenagers, and adults to cope better with everyday living with epilepsy.

Children with epilepsy may find that special recreation programs and summer camps help them to cope with seizures and medication and to deal with occasional discrimination. Peer support is especially important in adolescence.

Respite care programs offer families the opportunity for free time away from a child with a disability. Community agencies and affiliates of the Epilepsy Foundation can provide information about these programs.

It is important for parents to inform their child's teacher about the child's condition; how epilepsy affects the child; and what to do if a seizure occurs. Medication may slow the child's functional level. Children who have both epilepsy and learning disabilities or mental retardation will require special education services.

EPILEPSY IN ELDERS

There are about 300,000 cases of active epilepsy in the population over age 65 worldwide (Hauser and Hesdorffer: 1990). Seizures in elders may be the result of systemic illness; the use of medications such as analgesics and antihistamines; or the withdrawal of sedative drugs. Stroke, which occurs most frequently in elders, significantly increases an individual's risk of developing epilepsy.

It is crucial to identify any primary medical conditions that may precipitate seizures. Examples of systemic illnesses which may cause seizure activity include strokes (which may cause acute seizures followed by recurring seizure activity) and either primary or metastatic brain tumors. Once seizures symptomatic of systemic illness have been distinguished from epilepsy, they should be treated by managing the precipitating event without the use of anticonvulsant drugs (Troupin and Johannessen: 1990).

Individuals with chronic epilepsy may be affected by pharmacologic changes, such as changes in metabolism related to the aging process, and may require adjustment in their usual seizure therapy. Because elders often take drugs for a variety of conditions, elders with epilepsy must be concerned about the interaction of these drugs and anticonvulsants.

PSYCHOLOGICAL ASPECTS OF EPILEPSY

A recent study reported that individuals with epilepsy want to know what the condition is; what is happening to their bodies; what might happen in the future; and how they can better manage epilepsy (Schneider and Conrad: 1983). Knowledge and understanding were identified as the resources that enable individuals to deal better with epilepsy. Patients want their caregivers to listen to their fears and help them to adapt to life with epilepsy.

Individuals with epilepsy often find that aspects of everyday life are affected by their physical condition. Masland (1985) found that disability in individuals with epilepsy was related to the disruption caused by the seizures; the effects of associated neurological impairments, including those caused by drugs; reactions of society; and the individual's self-concept.

Unemployment and underemployment are among the most serious social problems of individuals with epilepsy. Although unpredictable seizures are hazardous in certain environments, they are less significant than the ignorance and fear of employers and employees. Employers must understand that medications may reduce productivity. In addition, poor self-image may have a negative effect on job-seeking skills and interpersonal relationships.

The lack of a driver's license can be a significant barrier to employment, activities of everyday living, and social life for the individual with epilepsy. In most states, an individual must be free of seizures for six months to one year in order to be eligible for a driver's license.

126

A letter from a physician which states that seizures are under control may be required.

It is often difficult for individuals with epilepsy to purchase health, life, or automobile insurance. Even when insurance is available, the premiums may be very high or exclusions may be made for claims relating to epilepsy.

Individuals whose seizures are under control have no restrictions on their recreational activities. However, it is important to take extra precautions with activities such as swimming, waterskiing, scuba, and sky diving, since the occurrence of a seizure is very dangerous while engaged in these activities. It is a good idea for individuals to wear an identification bracelet or necklace or carry a wallet card which indicates that they have epilepsy.

Depression in individuals with epilepsy may be due to the stresses of living with epilepsy; employment problems; or the inability to drive. An individual may complain of fatigue or feeling sad; may sleep poorly; or may be unable to concentrate. These symptoms may be related to having epilepsy, or they may signal a problem with medication. Participating in a self-help group, discussing these feelings with the physician, and using stress reduction and relaxation techniques may be helpful.

PROFESSIONAL SERVICE PROVIDERS

Individuals with epilepsy may receive treatment from a neurologist, pediatric neurologist, pediatrician, or a family physician.

Individuals who experience a seizure first see their *primary care physician*, either a family physician or a pediatrician. Hospitalization may be required to observe the patient for progressive symptoms or additional seizures. An out-patient visit may be sufficient if the seizure occurred more than a week before medical consultation and was an isolated event. The primary care physician may initiate treatment at this time.

If initial treatment does not achieve seizure control in about three months, the individual should be referred to a *neurologist* for a thorough evaluation. A neurologist is a physician who diagnoses and treats conditions involving the brain and nervous system, including epilepsy. A neurological assessment will include a patient history, physical examination, electroencephalograms (EEG), computerized tomography (CT) scan, magnetic resonance imaging (MRI), and other tests. If seizures are under control, the neurologist will follow the patient on an out-patient basis.

If seizures are not under control within nine months of treatment, referral to a comprehensive treatment center is recommended. The National Association of Epilepsy Centers has established guidelines for these specialized epilepsy treatment centers (Gumnit: 1990).

A *rehabilitation counselor* coordinates services such as vocational rehabilitation, education, and training for individuals with epilepsy. The rehabilitation counselor can serve as an advocate with prospective employers who may be uninformed or fearful about hiring an individual with epilepsy. Individuals with epilepsy who are unemployed or underemployed should apply to their state vocational rehabilitation agency for assistance with career planning, training, and placement.

WHERE TO FIND SERVICES

Physicians who treat people with epilepsy are often located in private practices. Individuals who live in metropolitan areas will find neurological clinics and comprehensive epilepsy centers available at major hospitals or universities. Comprehensive epilepsy centers and programs around the country provide medical care; conduct multidisciplinary research; train physicians, nurses and other caregivers; and help to organize community services. They are usually affiliated with university medical centers and serve a designated geographic area.

HOW TO RECOGNIZE A SEIZURE AND GIVE FIRST AID

Epileptic seizures have been mistakenly identified as heart attacks, drunkenness, and drug overdoses. It is important for all health professionals, rehabilitation professionals and the general public to recognize epileptic seizures and to know simple first aid for epilepsy.

- Remove hard or sharp items that are in the vicinity of the individual having a seizure.

- Loosen the individual's tie or collar to make breathing easier.

- Place a flat, soft cushion, folded jacket, or sweater under the individual's head.

- Gently turn the individual's head to the side to help keep the airway clear. Never try to place any object between the teeth of an individual experiencing a seizure.

- Do not try to stop the individual's jerking movements.

- Check to see if the individual is wearing an identification bracelet or necklace or carrying an identification card which states that he or she has epilepsy.

- Remain with the individual until the seizure ends and offer assistance, if needed.

128

• If the individual seems confused, offer to call a friend, family member, or taxi to help him/her get home.

• If the seizure continues for more than five minutes; if another seizure begins shortly after the first; or if the individual does not regain consciousness after the jerking movements have ceased, call an ambulance.

• If the individual is having an absence seizure, he or she may have a dazed appearance; stare into space; or exhibit automatic behavior such as shaking an arm or leg. Speak quietly and calmly and move the person away from any dangerous areas, such as a flight of stairs or a stove. Remain with the individual until consciousness returns.

References

Epilepsy Foundation of America
1990 <u>Medicines for Epilepsy</u> Landover, MD: Epilepsy Foundation of America
1989 <u>Questions and Answers About Epilepsy</u> Landover, MD: Epilepsy Foundation of America
1986 <u>A Patient's Guide to Medical Treatment of Childhood and Adult Seizure Disorders</u> Landover, MD: Epilepsy Foundation of America

Gumnit, Robert J.
1990 "Interplay of Economics, Politics, and Quality in the Care of Patients with Epilepsy: The Formation of the National Association of Epilepsy Centers" Appendix I in Dennis B. Smith (ed.) <u>Epilepsy: Current Approaches to Diagnosis and Treatment</u> New York: Raven Press

Hauser, W. Allen and Dale C. Hesdorffer
1990 <u>Facts About Epilepsy</u> Landover, MD: Epilepsy Foundation of America

Masland, R.L.
1985 "Psychosocial Aspects of Epilepsy" pp. 357-377 in Roger J. Porter (ed.) <u>The Epilepsies</u> Stoneham, MA: Butterworths

National Center on Health Statistics, Collins, John G.
1988 "Prevalence of Selected Chronic Conditions, United States, 1983-85" <u>Advance Data From Vital and Health Statistics</u> No. 155 DHHS Pub. No (PHS) 88-1250. Public Health Service. Hyattsville, MD

National Institute of Neurological Disorders and Stroke
1988 <u>The Surgical Management of Epilepsy</u> Bethesda, MD: National Institute of Neurological Disorders and Stroke

Schneider, Joseph W. and Peter Conrad
1983 Having Epilepsy: The Experience and Control of Illness   Philadelphia: Temple
      University Press

Smith, Dennis B.
1990 "Antiepileptic Drug Selection in Adults" pp. 111-138 in Dennis B. Smith (ed.) Epilepsy:
      Current Approaches to Diagnosis and Treatment New York: Raven Press

Troupin, Alan S and Svein I. Johannessen
1990 "Epilepsy in the Elderly" pp. 141-153 in Dennis B. Smith (ed.) Epilepsy: Current
      Approaches to Diagnosis and Treatment New York: Raven Press

Tyler, Allen R.
1990 "The Role of Surgery in Therapy for Epilepsy" pp. 173-182 in Dennis B. Smith (ed.)
      Epilepsy: Current Approaches to Diagnosis and Treatment New York: Raven Press

ORGANIZATIONS

(In the listings below, telephone numbers have symbols V for voice and TDD for tele-communication device for the deaf where organizations have published this information.)

Epilepsy Foundation of America (EFA)
4351 Garden City Drive, Suite 406
Landover, MD 20785
(800) 332-1000   (301) 459-3700

Provides information and education, advocacy, research support, and services to individuals with epilepsy, families, and professionals. Local affiliates. Some publications and audio-visual materials also available in Spanish. Benefits to EFA members include low-cost medication program and free monthly newsletter, "National Spokesman." Membership, $20.00; $5.00 limited membership provides eligibility for prescription drug program only.

National Association of Epilepsy Centers (NAEC)
5775 Wayzata Boulevard, Suite 225
Minneapolis, MN 55416
(612) 525-1160

An organization of epilepsy centers which helps to develop standards for medical and surgical treatment of epilepsy and for the facilities and programs which serve individuals with epilepsy. The NAEC also advises government and industry officials about the needs of people with epilepsy and offers technical assistance to the centers serving these individuals.

National Easter Seal Society
70 East Lake Street
Chicago, IL 60601
(312) 726-6200   (312) 726-4258 (TDD)

Provides information and services to individuals with epilepsy, their families, and professionals. Local affiliates.

National Epilepsy Library
Epilepsy Foundation of America (EFA)
4351 Garden City Drive
Landover, MD 20785
(800) 332-4050   (301) 459-3700

A professional library for physicians and other health professionals. Maintains database of articles and publications on medical and psychosocial aspects of epilepsy. Distributes "Quarterly Update," a bibliography of newly acquired resources, free.

131

National Head Injury Foundation (NHIF)
333 Turnpike Road
Southboro, MA 01772
(800) 444-6443   (508) 485-9950

A membership organization that provides information and support for individuals with head injury, their families, and professionals. (Epilepsy is often caused by a head injury.) Local affiliates. Membership fee of $35.00 includes quarterly "NHIF Newsletter." Also publishes the "National Directory of Head-Injury Rehabilitation Services." Members, $21.95; nonmembers, $32.95.

National Institute of Neurological Disorders and Stroke (NINDS)
Office of Scientific and Health Reports
Epilepsy Branch
National Institute of Health
Building 31, Room 8A-06
Bethesda, MD 20205
(301) 496-5751

Supports research, maintains national specimen banks for the study of brain and other tissue, and publishes professional and public education materials.

<u>As If By a Stroke of Lightening</u>
Altschul Group Corporation
930 Pitner Avenue .
Evanston, IL 60202
(800) 421-2363   (708) 328-6700

This videotape describes the causes and diagnosis of epilepsy, seizure types, and what to do when an individual has a seizure. $125.00

<u>Children with Epilepsy: A Parents' Guide</u>
by Helen Reisner (ed.)
Woodbine House
5615 Fishers Lane
Rockville, MD 20852

Discusses the diagnosis of epilepsy, treatment options, special education and legal rights, and coping strategies for children and their families. $14.95

<u>Epilepsy and the Family</u>
by Richard Lechtenberg
Harvard University Press, Cambridge, MA

In addition to basic information on epilepsy, this book includes chapters on children growing up with a parent who has epilepsy and on siblings and the extended family of individuals with epilepsy. Hardcover, $19.95; softcover, $8.95

<u>Epilepsy: You and Your Child</u>
Epilepsy Foundation of America (EFA)
4351 Garden City Drive
Landover, MD 20785
(800) 332-1000   (301) 459-3700

Designed to answer basic questions about epilepsy, this guide for parents also discusses psychosocial issues such as parental expectations, family dynamics, and interpersonal relationships as well as practical advice about school, special care, and resources. Free

<u>Family Video Library</u>
Epilepsy Foundation of America (EFA)
4351 Garden City Drive
Landover, MD 20785
(800) 332-1000   (301) 459-3700

This collection of videotapes is available for rental or sale. Includes subjects such as "Understanding Seizure Disorders," " How Medicines Work," "Epilepsy and the Family," "Living with Epilepsy," "Understanding Partial Seizures," "Epilepsy in the Teen Years," and "Epilepsy: The Child and the Family." Rental price is $10.00 per 3 day period, including one-way postage; purchase prices vary. Request a "Materials Service Center Catalog," free.

First Aid for Seizures
Epilepsy Foundation of America (EFA)
4351 Garden City Drive
Landover, MD 20785
(800) 332-1000   (301) 459-3700

Printed in both English and Spanish, this poster gives simple first aid instruction for people experiencing a seizure. Free

Living with Epilepsy
by Margaret Walker Sullivan
Bubba Press
2100 Cactus Court, #2
Walnut Creek, CA 94595

Written by a counselor who has epilepsy, this book provides practical advice for everyday living and discusses medical and psychosocial aspects of living with epilepsy. $6.95 plus $1.00 shipping and handling.

Room To Grow
CIBA-GEIGY Pharmaceuticals
556 Morris Avenue
Summit, NJ 07901
(800) 631-7994   (201) 277-5000, ext. 7361

Brochure which provides guidelines for parents of children with epilepsy. Includes helpful hints for babysitters and suggestions for discipline and other child development issues. Free

Seizures and Epilepsy in Childhood: A Guide for Parents
by John M. Freeman, Eileen P.G. Vining, and Diana J. Pillas
Johns Hopkins, Baltimore, MD

Describes how seizures occur, diagnostic tests, medication, surgery, and social implications of epilepsy. $18.95

<u>Trick Or Treat Or Trouble</u>
by Barbara Aiello and Jeffrey Shulman
9385-C Gerwig Lane
Columbia, MD 21046
(800) 368-5437   (301) 290-9095

One of the "Kids on the Block" series, this book on epilepsy is written for children in grades two to five. $12.95

LOW BACK PAIN

Low back pain is one of the most prevalent debilitating conditions in North America. A recent study found that back pain (both lower and upper) was the most common type of pain presented by patients whose primary reason for visiting physicians' offices was pain that lasted at least three months (National Center for Health Statistics: 1986). Low back pain occurs most frequently in people in the middle age range. Occupations that involve heavy lifting and other chronic repetitive movements have a clear relation with the incidence of low back pain (Vermont Rehabilitation Engineering Center: no date). People whose work requires that they sit in the same position for extended periods of time are also prone to low back pain; for example, it is known that truck drivers have a high rate of low back pain.

THE BACK

The back has three main components, the *vertebrae*, the *disks*, and a *network of ligaments*. Each vertebra has two main parts, the anterior body consisting of bone, and the posterior arch, a thick bony hollow structure, through which the spinal cord passes. The 33 bony, interlocking vertebrae include seven cervical or neck vertebrae, 12 thoracic or high back vertebrae, five lumbar or low back vertebrae, five sacral vertebrae near the base of the spine, and four coccygeal vertebrae fused to form the coccyx. The higher vertebrae are larger than the lower vertebrae and therefore are stronger and able to withstand greater stress. Between each pair of vertebrae are disks, soft tissues made up largely of gelatinous substance and water. Intervertebral disks act as cushions to absorb the shock of motion. Cartilage and fiber between the disks, called nucleus pulposus, absorb shocks and strains. Joints lined with cartilage along the vertebral arch are called facets. The spinal cord, consisting of a narrow bundle of nerve cells and fibers, runs from the base of the brain through the hollow structure of the vertebrae. The brain's communication with the rest of the body is carried out through these nerve fibers. Smaller bundles of nerves branch out between each pair of vertebrae. These secondary nerve cells are called nerve roots (American Medical Association: 1982).

The lumbar, or lower region of the back, supports most of the torso and is susceptible to great stress. It is for this reason that most back problems occur in the lower or lumbar region. Low back pain may be caused by a variety of factors, including diseases such as osteoarthritis, osteoporosis, and gynecological disorders and injuries incurred by twisting, bending, or lifting. Both too much exercise and too little exercise have been cited as causes of low back pain. Emotional stress, which causes muscle tension, has also been implicated as a causal factor. The normal aging process causes the disks to dry out and grow thinner; however, older people are less likely to have back pain than younger people, probably because they are less likely to be engaged in occupations that require lifting or repetitive movements.

NONSPECIFIC LOW BACK PAIN

Most low back pain is "nonspecific," since the cause is not known; the usual diagnosis is a sprained or strained back. Although most people with back pain will recover in three months or less, some people experience chronic, persistent back pain. For these individuals, chronic low back pain may alter their entire lifestyle, requiring time away from work and assistance with daily activities and household tasks.

In the first episode of nonspecific low back pain, the usual treatment is a combination of *bed rest, aspirin*, and perhaps the short term use of a *muscle relaxant*. Patients who are overweight; whose occupations predispose them to back pain; or who do not exercise may be advised to lose weight and begin a program of exercise when the pain subsides (Public Health Service: 1989). Although exercise is frequently prescribed, there is little scientific evidence to validate its effectiveness. Analgesics are prescribed in just under half of all visits to physicians for back pain. Psychotropic drugs, defined as antianxiety agents, sedatives, antidepressants, and antipsychotic drugs, are prescribed in only 13% of all office visits for back pain (National Center for Health Statistics: 1986).

The application of *heat*, in the form of hot water bottles or electrical heating pads, is sometimes prescribed, although the heat does not penetrate deeply enough to reach the affected tissues. Infra-red heat, or heat lamps, may be more effective because the wave lengths are able to penetrate the skin (Jayson: 1981).

A variety of other treatments are prescribed for people with chronic back pain, although the benefit of many of these treatments is either unproven or controversial. *Surgery* is considered in only a small proportion of all cases. Even in cases of chronic back pain, there is usually no evidence of a physical condition that can be remedied by surgery (Frymoyer: 1988).

Transcutaneous electric nerve stimulation (TENS) is a treatment method in which low level electric impulses are delivered to nerve endings under the skin near the source of pain. It is not known why TENS should alleviate pain, and a recent study found that patients with low back pain who received TENS treatment did not improve significantly more than the control group members, who received a "sham" treatment (Deyo et al.: 1990)

Traction, a treatment that involves the positioning of weights attached to pulleys, which are in turn tied to bandages on the legs, may produce short term improvement. However, recent studies suggest that traction may be effective only because it requires that the patient stay in bed (Frymoyer: 1988), thereby decreasing the probability of further injury to damaged nerves and ligaments.

Manipulation is a method of treatment that uses the hands to bend, twist, or stretch stiff joints and to relieve muscles spasms. It is not possible to manipulate bones, however (Hall: 1980). Although some studies suggest a temporary benefit of short term manipulation, there is little evidence to indicate that it has lasting benefits or that long term manipulation is effective (Frymoyer: 1988).

Work hardening is an individualized rehabilitation plan in which the person performs tasks that are part of his or her occupation. The individual is taught to build up muscle strength and to carry out the work tasks in a safe and efficient way without causing damage to the body. Although the individual's capacity and endurance may be limited at first, the goal is to build up to the optimal capacity needed to perform the tasks without overloading the body.

OTHER TYPES OF BACK PAIN

Prolapsed intervertebral disks are disks which have ruptured or burst (often incorrectly referred to as "slipped disks"). Disks may herniate or rupture because of weakening of the disks themselves or of intervertebral cartilage; excessive strain; or an injury. It is possible for any disk to burst, but ruptures occur most frequently in the lower back or the lumbar region, since this area is subject to the greatest stress. Disks that are likely to burst are those that have already degenerated or have cracks; when the stress is too great for these disks, they may burst or rupture. Although disks themselves have no nerves, when they burst, fragments of the disk may press on ligaments and nerves nearby, causing pain. The pain caused by the pressure of disk fragments on a nerve is often referred to as a pinched nerve.

In some individuals, stiffness may precede the pain of a ruptured disk. In other cases, severe pain is very sudden, and the individual may be unable to stand erect. This pain is called *acute lumbago* (Jayson: 1981). Treatment for ruptured disks usually involves bed rest for several weeks on a firm bed with a board underneath to prevent the mattress from sagging. Bed rest is beneficial because it prevents movement and rubbing of the inflamed tissues, which exacerbate the pain. Surgery is usually not necessary; when surgery is performed, fragments of the ruptured disk and the remaining part of the disk that may potentially rupture are removed.

Sciatica involves pain along the sciatic nerve, which extends from the base of the spine to the thigh, with branches throughout the legs and feet. Sciatica may be caused by inflammation; toxicity such as lead or alcohol poisoning; injury to a disk; arthritis; or pressure on a nerve. Diagnosis of sciatica requires repeated physical examinations. Most patients recover from sciatica in six weeks or less, suggesting that surgery is warranted only in severe cases and in cases where a tumor, ruptured disk, or epidural abscess is present (Frymoyer: 1988; Jayson: 1981).

Ankylosing spondylitis is a stiffening of the spine that may be so severe that it results in the total loss of motion in the back. The person with ankylosing spondylitis may appear extremely round shouldered with a stoop in the upper back. Ankylosing spondylitis occurs most frequently in men age 15 to 25. Treatment includes physiotherapy and correction of posture (Jayson: 1981).

Rheumatoid arthritis is a chronic condition which causes inflammation of the joints of the body, including those of the spine. Its onset is usually in midlife, although it may also occur in children and elders. Rheumatoid arthritis subsides and recurs and may cause severe disability. Rheumatoid arthritis can also cause general weakness, fatigue, and loss of appetite. Rheumatoid arthritis affects two million Americans and twice as many women as men (National Institute of Arthritis and Musculoskeletal and Skin Diseases: 1987).

Osteoarthritis is a noninflammatory condition in which the cartilage, the material that protects the end of bones and other joints, ulcerates, frays, or degenerates. It may occur in a single joint due to an injury or infection. Osteoarthritis is most common among elders. More than 16 million Americans are affected by osteoarthritis (National Institute of Arthritis and Musculoskeletal and Skin Diseases: 1987).

PSYCHOLOGICAL ASPECTS OF LOW BACK PAIN

Although many observers have suggested that psychological characteristics such as neurosis are related to low back pain, it is not clear whether the low back pain causes these psychological characteristics or vice versa. Certainly, individuals who experience unremitting pain are likely to have intense emotional responses. Since the most common treatment for back pain is bed rest, individuals with back pain find themselves isolated, unable to work, and unable to carry out the minimal requirements of daily living. When analgesics and sedatives are prescribed and used over a period of time, they can have effects on the individual's moods and behavior; therefore, most physicians prescribe these drugs for use on a short term basis only.

The inability to work causes financial problems for most individuals, resulting in increased tension and anxiety. Vocational rehabilitation counselors can help individuals who are unable to continue with their usual work to seek out alternative employment and financial compensation to bridge the gap between positions.

Back pain also interferes with normal sexual activity, causing additional strain in marital relations. People who have experienced low back pain in the past may fear that sexual intercourse will precipitate another attack. Back schools (described below), pain clinics, and self-help groups teach individuals techniques that decrease stress on the back and concomitantly decrease anxiety associated with sexual intercourse.

Methods of alleviating tension, which may contribute to back pain in the form of tense muscles, may reduce anxiety and help people feel that they are in control of their own lives. Relaxation techniques and meditation are frequently used to help people with back pain to relieve tension. Behavior modification has the goal of changing the individual's lifestyle by increasing mobility and independence.

Pain clinics are one source of help for people who experience chronic low back pain. More than 800 pain clinics in the United States are settings where a multidisciplinary team of health care providers design an individualized treatment plan for each patient. A variety of treatment modalities are used for each patient, including exercise, diet modification, transcutaneous electric nerve stimulation, individual or group psychotherapy, massage, and analgesic medications.

Back school is a term that has been adopted recently to indicate a multifaceted treatment approach with an emphasis on patient education. Patients learn about anatomy; proper seating, posture and lifting; and exercise regimens. In addition, many back schools offer psychological counseling and training in stress management (Carron and Tanenbaum: 1987). Back schools may be operated by physical therapists in private practice or in other medical settings.

In some cases, it may be necessary for employees with low back pain to be trained to obtain positions that are less physically demanding than their previous positions. Both state and private rehabilitation agencies provide services that enable people with chronic back pain to obtain or retain employment (see Appendix A for a list of state vocational rehabilitation agencies). Many programs either sponsored or funded by the government are available to train people with disabilities for productive employment (See <u>Meeting the Needs of Employees with Disabilities</u>, described in "PUBLICATIONS AND TAPES" section below for a more detailed description of these programs.) In some instances, insurance companies pay for the cost of these programs. Because back problems are frequently a result of injuries incurred on the job, some large employers also have in-house rehabilitation programs to enable employees to return to their previous position or to positions with modified work tasks.

Self-help groups enable people with low back pain to discuss their problems with others who may have similar situations; to share solutions to common problems; and to express their emotional responses to chronic pain. Several organizations (see "ORGANIZATIONS" section below) refer individuals to appropriate self-help groups in their own geographic area.

PROFESSIONAL SERVICE PROVIDERS

Most people who have back pain begin the search for treatment with their *family physician*, *general practitioner*, or *internist,* who may prescribe bed rest and analgesics. If a condition that requires special treatment is suspected, the family physician may refer the patient to a specialist.

Osteopaths are doctors whose training emphasizes the musculoskeletal system. *Orthopedists* or *orthopedic surgeons* specialize in diseases of the musculoskeletal system. When nerve involvement is suspected, *neurologists* will evaluate the patient to determine the exact location of the problem. *Rheumatologists* are physicians who specialize in rheumatic diseases such as osteoarthritis. *Physiatrists* are physicians who specialize in rehabilitation medicine and work closely with physical therapists.

After examining patients with low back pain, physicians may refer patients to *physical therapists*, who will evaluate the physical condition and the dysfunction it causes and prescribe traction, manipulation, heat or cold therapy, exercise, or massage. Some physical therapists work in hospitals or rehabilitation centers, while others are in private practice. *Chiropractors* treat back problems through a procedure called manipulation, which involves exerting pressure on joints or muscles.

Vocational rehabilitation counselors assess the situation of individuals with low back pain; place them in training programs, if necessary; work with employers to arrange for modification of positions or job sharing; and place clients in appropriate positions.

MODIFICATIONS IN DAILY LIVING

Suggestions for prevention of low back pain include the following:

• Modify the environment both in the home and the workplace so that chairs, work surfaces, beds, and driver's seats provide support for the back. For example, chairs should be well padded but not overly stuffed and should have a firm back. Beds should be firm, possibly shored up with a board underneath the mattress. Special back supports and cushions help some people feel more comfortable. These items are available in a number of health care product mail order catalogues (see Chapter 4, "Making Everyday Living Easier") as well as in retail stores.

• Long periods of sitting in one position should be avoided. If it is necessary to remain in one position for a prolonged period of time, there should be periodic breaks of moving around.

• Obesity causes an additional strain on the back; therefore, people who are overweight should strive to lose excess pounds.

• Many experts suggest regular exercise. Swimming, walking, and exercises such as sit-ups to strengthen the abdominal muscles are recommended. Individuals with specific back problems should consult the appropriate professional service provider to design a special exercise program to meet their needs.

• Heavy objects should be lifted by bending the legs and keeping the back straight.

• Poor posture, which is thought to be one possible cause of back pain, should be improved. Care should be taken to ensure that the buttocks do not protrude, as this causes the lower back to arch in an abnormal position.

No matter what the cause or condition, experts who treat people with low back pain all agree that early intervention is crucial. The longer that individuals with low back pain remain incapacitated and away from their work, the less likely it is that they will return.

References

American Medical Association
1982 Book of Back Care New York: Random House

Carron, Harold, and Richard L. Tanenbaum
1987 Rehabilitation of Persons with Chronic Low Back Pain Washington DC: D:ATA Institute, Catholic University of America

Deyo, Richard A., Nicolas E. Walsh, Donald C. Martin, Lawrence S. Schoenfeld, and Somayajo Ramamurthy
1990 "A Controlled Trial of Transcutaneous Electrical Nerve Stimulation (TENS) and Exercise for Chronic Low Back Pain" New England Journal of Medicine 322(June 7):23:1627-1634

Frymoyer, John W.
1988 "Back Pain and Sciatica" New England Journal of Medicine 318(Feb 4):5:291-300

Frymoyer, John W. and William Cats-Baril
1987 "Predictors of Low Back Pain Disability" Clinical Orthopaedics 221(August):89-98

Hall, Hamilton
1980 The Back Doctor New York: McGraw-Hill

Jayson, Malcolm
1981 Back Pain: The Facts New York: Oxford University Press

National Center for Health Statistics, Koch, H.
1986 "The Management of Chronic Pain in Office-Based Ambulatory Care: National Ambulatory Medical Care Survey Advance Data from Vital and Health Statistics No. 123, DHHS Pub. No. (PHS) 86-1250 Public Health Service Hyattsville, MD

National Institute of Arthritis and Musculoskeletal and Skin Diseases
1987 Arthritis, Rheumatic diseases, and Related Disorders Public Health Service

Public Health Service
1989 <u>Chronic Pain Hope through Research</u> NIH Publication No. 90-2406

Vermont Rehabilitation Engineering Center
no date   "Biomechanics and Low Back Pain" <u>REC Brief</u>, 1:1:1-10

(In the listings below, telephone numbers have symbols V for voice and TDD for tele-communication device for the deaf where organizations have published this information.)

<u>American Back Society</u> (ABS)
St. Joseph's Professional Center
2647 East 14th Street, Suite 401
Oakland, CA 94601
(415) 536-9929

A membership organization dedicated to relieving the pain and impairment caused by back problems. Sponsors symposia for presenting research findings. Membership for licensed health care professionals, $200.00; for other interested individuals, $100.00. Publishes quarterly "ABS Newsletter," which is a benefit of membership, or it may be purchased for $35.00 per year.

<u>American Chronic Pain Association</u> (ACPA)
PO Box 850
Rocklin, CA 95677
(916) 632-0922

Organizes groups throughout the United States and Canada to provide support and activities for people who experience chronic pain. Individual lay membership, free; professional membership, $50.00. Publishes quarterly newsletter, "ACPA Chronicle," $5.00.

<u>The Arthritis Foundation</u>
1314 Spring Street, NW
Atlanta, GA 30309
(800) 283-7800   (404) 872-7100

Supports research; offers referrals to physicians; provides public and professional education; and offers a discount drug service. Chapters throughout the United States. Some chapters offer arthritis classes, clubs, and exercise programs. Membership fee of $20.00, includes chapter newsletter and magazine, "Arthritis Today."

<u>The Arthritis Society</u>
250 Bloor Street East, Suite 401
Toronto, Ontario M4W 3P2 Canada
(416) 947-1414

Supports research and medical training programs; provides information and educational materials; and conducts self-help groups. Publishes "Arthritis News" and "Communique" (in French). Subscription, $10.00

National Arthritis and Musculoskeletal and Skin Diseases Information Clearinghouse
Box AMS
Bethesda, MD 20892
(301) 495-4484

Compiles and distributes information to health care professionals through a data base. Distributes bibliographies, fact sheets, catalogues, and directories. Requests from individuals are referred to the Arthritis Foundation.

National Chronic Pain Outreach Association (NCPOA)
7979 Old Georgetown Road, Suite 100
Bethesda, MD 20814-2429
(301) 652-4948

A national clearinghouse for information about chronic pain. Refers individuals to support groups on chronic pain throughout the United States and Canada. Produces publications and cassettes on a variety of topics related to chronic pain. Individual membership of $25.00 includes quarterly newsletter, "Lifeline."

National Institute of Arthritis and Musculoskeletal and Skin Diseases (NIAMSD)
Building 31, Room 4C-32B
9000 Rockville Pike
Bethesda, MD 20892
(301) 496-8188

NIAMSD sponsors specialized research centers in rheumatoid arthritis, osteoarthritis, and osteoporosis. These centers conduct basic and clinical research; provide professional, public, and patient education; and are involved in community activities. Also supports individual clinical and basic research.

Vermont Rehabilitation Engineering Center
1 South Prospect Street
Burlington, VT 05401
(800) 527-7320   (802) 656-4582

A federally funded research center that investigates prevention, assessment, and rehabilitation of low back pain. Maintains "Backfiles," a bibliographic database for both professionals and consumers. Publishes monographs and informational brochures as well as semi-annual "Rehab Briefs," $3.00 per copy.

Coping with Osteoarthritis and
Coping with Rheumatoid Arthritis
both by Robert H. Phillips
Avery Publishing, Garden City, NY

Each book discusses strategies for improving the quality of life. Each has sections on working, pain, exercise and rest. $9.95 each

Directory of Pain Management Facilities
American Pain Society
PO Box 186
Skokie, IL 60076-0186

A listing of pain management facilities. $30.00

Guide to Independent Living for People with Arthritis
Arthritis Foundation
1314 Spring Street, NW
Atlanta, GA 30309
(800) 283-7800   (404) 872-7100

Describes self-help aids, product manufacturers, distributors, and mail order firms. Includes categories such as posture and transfer, mobility aids, grooming, dressing, and service groups. Available through local affiliates of the Arthritis Foundation only; call the Foundation's National Office to request information on your local affiliate.

Living with Arthritis
Resources for Rehabilitation
33 Bedford Street, Suite 19A
Lexington, MA 02173
(617) 862-6455

One title in a series of large print publications designed for distribution by professionals to people with disabilities. Includes information on how to obtain services, organizations that serve people with arthritis, publications, and aids that help people with arthritis. Minimum purchase 25 copies. $2.00 per copy See order form opposite inside back cover.

Meeting the Needs of Employees with Disabilities
Resources for Rehabilitation
33 Bedford Street, Suite 19A
Lexington, MA 02173
(617) 862-6455

Provides information to help people with disabilities retain or obtain employment. Information on government programs and laws, supported employment, training programs, environmental adaptations, and the transition from school to work are included. Chapters on mobility, vision, and hearing and speech impairments include information on organizations, products, and services that enable employers to accommodate the needs of employees with disabilities. $42.95 plus $5.00 shipping and handling.

Understand Your Backache
by Rene Cailliet
F.A. Davis, Philadelphia, PA

Includes information about treatment and prevention of back pain as well as a description of the examinations performed by physicians and various types of surgery. $11.95

MULTIPLE SCLEROSIS

Multiple sclerosis (MS) is a chronic central nervous system condition in which the nerve fibers of the brain and spinal cord are damaged. A fatty substance called myelin protects the nerve fibers and enables the smooth transmission of neurological impulses between the central nervous system and the rest of the body. If inflammation damages or destroys the myelin, it may heal with no loss of function. Later, however, scar (or plaque) may form and interfere with the transmission of neurological impulses. Function is diminished or lost. The disease is called multiple sclerosis because there are multiple areas of scarring or sclerosis (Minden and Frankel: 1989).

Estimates of individuals with multiple sclerosis vary from less than 200,000, based on hospital and physicians' records, to a half million, based on public surveys and pathology records (National Institute of Neurological Disorders and Stroke: 1990). Multiple sclerosis affects twice as many women as men and twice as many whites as blacks (Scheinberg and Smith: 1989). Age of onset ranges from mid to late adolescence to middle age.

Multiple sclerosis can cause severe disability in individuals in their most productive years (National Multiple Sclerosis Society: 1989). Nearly 77% of individuals with multiple sclerosis have activity limitations (National Center on Health Statistics: 1988). The broad economic and social implications of multiple sclerosis include medical expenses, unemployment or underemployment, the cost of special services, and the emotional and physical effects on the individual as well as the family.

Each person with multiple sclerosis has unique symptoms based on the location of the damage to the nervous system. These symptoms may include blurred or double vision, numbness in the extremities, balance or coordination problems, fatigue, muscle spasticity or stiffness, slurred speech, muscle weakness, or loss of bladder or bowel control.

The cause of multiple sclerosis is unknown. Scientists who believe that multiple sclerosis is an autoimmune disease are investigating the role of a variety of viruses in triggering damage to the immune system, which in turn may lead to the development of multiple sclerosis (National Institute of Neurological Disorders and Stroke: no date). Other investigators are studying the role of heredity. Their studies suggest that certain genetic factors may predispose some individuals to acquire multiple sclerosis, but there is no known pattern of direct inheritance.

DIAGNOSIS OF MULTIPLE SCLEROSIS

A positive diagnosis of multiple sclerosis may take months or years. Physicians must verify loss of function in more than one area of the central nervous system and confirm that these losses have occurred at least twice. Patients are often frustrated by the length of time and the multiple procedures required to diagnose their symptoms.

If the individual's medical history and physical examination do not confirm a positive diagnosis of multiple sclerosis, diagnostic procedures such as evoked potentials, computer tomography, and magnetic resonance imaging may be performed.

Evoked potentials (EP) measure how fast electrical impulses travel through the central nervous system to the brain. The physician may use one of three evoked potentials to assess various losses of function. The visual evoked potential assesses the visual pathway to the optic nerve; the somatosensory evoked potential studies sensory reactions and limb and spinal cord nerve function; and the brainstem auditory evoked potential may reveal the cause of hearing and balance problems. Evoked potentials are performed on an out-patient basis. Electrodes are placed on the skin, using a conducting ointment. A mild electrical stimulus is administered by the technician, and a computer records the brain's response to the stimulus. The physician studies the computer recordings to determine the site of neurological damage.

Computerized tomography (CT) scans use x-rays to scan the central nervous system for signs of demyelination. A dye is injected to provide contrast between normal and abnormal areas. Since the development of magnetic resonance imaging (MRI), CT scans have been used less frequently.

The MRI is considered to be nearly 90% accurate in diagnosing multiple sclerosis (Calvano: 1989). The MRI's images are produced by the interaction between its magnetic field and the hydrogen atoms which make up body cells. The MRI provides a recorded image of central nervous system lesions. Some of these lesions may be detected in the MRI before any symptoms appear or loss of function occurs. Because MRI's are so accurate, diagnostic procedures used in the past, such as lumbar punctures and myelography (an x-ray procedure), are now used infrequently.

TYPES OF MULTIPLE SCLEROSIS

Individuals with the *benign* form of multiple sclerosis experience little or no progression of the disease after the initial attack. The benign form affects about 20% of individuals with multiple sclerosis (Scheinberg: 1983). The most common symptoms are optic neuritis (inflammation of the optic nerve) and numbness of a limb. Individuals have no permanent disability.

Exacerbating-remitting describes a pattern of multiple sclerosis in which the individual experiences sudden deterioration followed by almost complete remission of symptoms. This pattern continues for months or years with few physical restrictions. About 25% of individuals have this form of multiple sclerosis (Scheinberg: 1983).

Individuals with the *chronic-relapsing* form of multiple sclerosis have remissions after exacerbations of the disease, but the cumulative effects of the symptoms slowly lead to disability. About 40% of individuals with multiple sclerosis experience this form of the disease.

The most severely disabling form of the disease is *chronic-progressive* multiple sclerosis, which occurs in about 15% of the population with multiple sclerosis (Scheinberg: 1983). In these individuals, the disease progresses without remission and may result in disability very quickly.

These forms of multiple sclerosis are not exclusive; some individuals may experience progression of one form to another. Smith and Scheinberg (1985) report that there is a more favorable prognosis for individuals with early onset (before age 35); acute onset rather than gradual onset; complete remission after the first attack; and sensory rather than motor symptoms.

TREATMENT OF MULTIPLE SCLEROSIS

There is no cure for multiple sclerosis; however, physicians can treat the symptoms of multiple sclerosis and try to control its progress with anti-inflammatory medication. Prednisone, ACTH (adrenocorticotropic hormone), prednisolone, and other anti-inflammatory drugs have been effective in reducing the severity and duration of multiple sclerosis attacks. These medications are not recommended for long-term use because of side effects such as nausea, drowsiness, changes in blood pressure and blood sugar levels, lowered resistance to infection, and thinning of bones (Lechtenberg: 1988).

Medication may also be used to treat multiple sclerosis symptoms such as spasticity, dizziness, fatigue, bladder problems, tremors, depression, and sensory problems, such as a "pins and needles" feeling. The individual with multiple sclerosis and the physician must carefully consider each medication and its possible side effects, which may appear to be symptoms of the disease itself.

Optic neuritis, *double vision*, and *nystagmus* are common visual symptoms of multiple sclerosis. Inflammation of the optic nerve (neuritis) causes loss of vision. If the muscles of the eye are weakened by nerve demyelination, the individual cannot focus and experiences double vision (diplopia). Double vision may occur during an exacerbation and disappear during remission of multiple sclerosis symptoms. Cortisone is often used to treat optic neuritis and double vision. Nystagmus is an involuntary rapid eye movement; it interferes with focusing and may cause dizziness.

Some individuals with multiple sclerosis experience ***problems with gait*** including weakness, spasticity, and lack of coordination (ataxia). Antispastic medications, stretching exercises, and swimming relieve symptoms such as a stiff gait, foot drop, and toe dragging. Orthoses are assistive devices used to support weakened areas, provide proper alignment, and improve function. An ankle foot orthosis worn inside the shoe may relieve the symptoms of spasticity. Ataxia is treated with a sequential exercise program in which the individual performs repetitive movements, often watching him or herself in a mirror, to increase sensory feedback and restore coordination.

Urinary, bowel, and ***sexual dysfunction***; ***weakness of upper extremities***; ***fatigue***; and ***speech problems*** (dysarthria) are other disabling symptoms of multiple sclerosis. Individuals with severe multiple sclerosis may also have difficulty swallowing. Treatment options for these symptoms include medication, exercise, adaptations in everyday living, and adjustment counseling.

PSYCHOLOGICAL ASPECTS OF MULTIPLE SCLEROSIS

The unpredictability of multiple sclerosis and the fact that individuals with the disease have a near-normal life expectancy (Scheinberg: 1983) require continual adjustment and re-adjustment. The unpredictability of exacerbations is very frustrating to individuals with multiple sclerosis. Individuals must plan their daily living and work schedules to accommodate the effects of the condition. For example, exacerbations often cause fatigue, which interferes with normal activities. Individuals must find a balance between activity and rest periods.

When making plans for living arrangements or for travel, individuals with multiple sclerosis must consider a variety of alternatives in the event that their functional abilities deteriorate. For instance, in purchasing a home, it is wise to determine if there is room for a wheelchair ramp.

Symptoms such as stumbling, dropping items, incontinence, and slurred speech may lead to self-consciousness, anxiety, and depression. The individual's personal coping mechanisms and the support provided by family, friends, and the community are crucial to the active problem-solving required in living with multiple sclerosis (Shuman and Schwartz: 1988). Individuals who exhibit these symptoms may also benefit from individual or group counseling.

PROFESSIONAL SERVICE PROVIDERS

The unique symptoms of each individual with multiple sclerosis require individualized treatment plans. The physical and emotional needs of each individual are best served through a team approach involving medical, allied health, and rehabilitation professionals.

Neurologists, who specialize in diseases and conditions of the brain and central nervous system, conduct neurological examinations and interpret the results of tests such as MRI's and CT scans to diagnose multiple sclerosis and to rule out other possible conditions. *Physiatrists,* or rehabilitation physicians, design an individual treatment plan for the patient with multiple sclerosis.

Physical therapists teach individuals with multiple sclerosis how to perform a range of exercises which help build endurance and strength. Physical therapists also prescribe therapeutic exercises to diminish or eliminate weakness, spasticity, and lack of coordination. Physical therapists train the individual to use assistive devices such as canes, crutches, and orthoses.

Occupational therapists assess functioning in activities of everyday living and teach simplified techniques of accomplishing them. They may recommend adaptations to the home and work environments. Occupational therapists also suggest adaptive recreation equipment and programs.

Orthotists make and fit assistive devices for improving gait in individuals with multiple sclerosis. A physical or occupational therapist teaches the individual how to use these devices, such as ankle or foot braces.

Rehabilitation nurses provide skilled nursing care; instruct patients and family members in proper patient care; do follow-up upon discharge from a hospital; and make referrals to community services.

Social workers offer practical and emotional support to individuals adjusting to a disability or chronic condition and to their families. Social workers provide information about financial and medical benefits, housing, and community resources. They conduct individual, family, or group counseling and may refer individuals to self-help or peer counseling groups.

WHERE TO FIND SERVICES

Neurologists are found in private practice, acute care hospitals, and specialty clinics. Local affiliates of the National Multiple Sclerosis Society may offer a referral service to neurologists who specialize in the treatment of multiple sclerosis. Neurologists and other members of the multidisciplinary team may also work in transitional or independent living programs and in rehabilitation hospitals. Some physical and occupational therapists may come to the patient's home to provide services.

ENVIRONMENTAL ADAPTATIONS

Individuals with multiple sclerosis use a combination of environmental adaptations and assistive devices to make everyday routines easier.

152

Some individuals with gait problems use a cane, crutches, walker, wheelchair, scooter, or a combination of these mobility aids. An individual who usually uses a cane or crutches may prefer to use a wheelchair or scooter when traveling long distances.

Heat and humidity affect many individuals with multiple sclerosis. Air conditioning helps to reduce fatigue and weakness. Individuals with multiple sclerosis should ask their physician, rehabilitation counselor, or tax adviser if the purchase of an air conditioner is a tax-deductible expense.

A referral to a low vision rehabilitation center offers individuals with vision problems the opportunity to improve visual function with low vision aids. An eye patch may reduce double vision. Prisms, mounted on the eyeglasses lens, will expand the visual field of the eye that is not patched. Sunglasses reduce glare and improve contrast for individuals with optic neuritis. Nonoptical aids such as large print, tape recorders, and high contrast markings are also useful assistive devices (see Chapter 11, "Visual Impairment and Blindness").

Bathtub rails, elevated toilet seats, and grab bars are useful bathroom safety devices. A stall shower is safer and easier to use than a combination tub/shower. A shower chair or tub seat provides additional safety.

Special controls installed on cars with automatic transmissions enable many individuals with multiple sclerosis to continue driving. The gas and brake pedals are operated by hand. These attachments do not interfere with the foot pedals used by other family members.

Some individuals use adaptive devices for dressing, including elastic shoelaces, velcro closures, and buttoning aids. Foam hair rollers, water pipe foam insulation, or layers of tape are used to build up the handles of items as varied as toothbrushes, pens, pencils, eating utensils, paint brushes, and crochet hooks.

Remote controls turn on and off lights and televisions and open and close garage doors. Voice dialer telephones allow the individual to store frequently called telephone numbers and to call them automatically. A speaker phone allows individuals with poor motor control or tremors to carry on a telephone conversation comfortably.

Individuals with multiple sclerosis can save time and energy by reorganizing the kitchen and changing food preparation routines. Many individuals learn valuable tips and techniques from peers in multiple sclerosis support groups or from occupational therapists.

Many mail order catalogs offer a wide selection of adaptive aids for individuals with disabilities and chronic conditions. (See Chapter 4, "Making Everyday Living Easier," for sources of these devices.)

References

Calvano, Margaret
1989 <u>Facts & Issues</u> New York, NY: National Multiple Sclerosis Society

Goldenson, Robert M.
1978 "Rehabilitation Professions" in Robert M. Goldenson (ed.) <u>Disability and Rehabilitation Handbook</u> New York: McGraw-Hill, Inc.

Holland, Nancy J., Phyllis Wiesel-Levison, and Michele G. Madonna
1984 "Community Care of the Patient with Multiple Sclerosis" <u>Rehabilitation Nursing</u> (Nov-Dec):18-20

Lechtenberg, Richard
1988 <u>Multiple Sclerosis Fact Book</u> Philadelphia: FA Davis Company

Minden, Sarah L. and Debra Frankel
1989 <u>PLAINTALK: A Booklet About Multiple Sclerosis For Family Members</u> New York, NY: National Multiple Sclerosis Society

National Center on Health Statistics, Collins, John G.
1988 "Prevalence of Selected Chronic Conditions, United States, 1983-85" <u>Advance Data From Vital and Health Statistics</u>. No. 155 DHHS Pub. No (PHS) 88-1250. Public Health Service. Hyattsville, MD

National Institute of Neurological Disorders and Stroke
No <u>Multiple Sclerosis: 1990 Research Program</u> Bethesda, MD: National Institutes of
date Health

Robbins, Kate and Arthur S. Abramson
1987 "Aids to Ease the Activities of Daily Living" pp. 91-110 in Labe C. Scheinberg (ed.) <u>Multiple Sclerosis: A Guide for Patients and Their Families</u> New York: Raven Press

Scheinberg, Labe
1983 "Signs, Symptoms, and Course of MS" pp. 35-43 in Labe C. Scheinberg (ed.) <u>Multiple Sclerosis: A Guide for Patients and Their Families</u> New York: Raven Press

Scheinberg, Labe and Charles R. Smith
1989 <u>Rehabilitation of Patients with Multiple Sclerosis</u> New York, NY: National Multiple Sclerosis Society

Shuman, Robert and Janice Schwartz
1988 <u>Understanding Multiple Sclerosis</u> Riverside, NJ: MacMillan Publishing Company

Smith, Charles R. and Labe Scheinberg

1990 "Symptomatic Treatment and Rehabilitation in Multiple Sclerosis" pp. 327-350 in Stuart D. Cook (ed.) <u>Handbook of Multiple Sclerosis</u> New York: Marcel Dekker, Inc.

1985 "Clinical Features of Multiple Sclerosis" <u>Seminars in Neurology</u> 5:(June)2:85-93

Wasserman, Lynn

1978 <u>Living with Multiple Sclerosis: A Practical Guide</u> New York, NY: National Multiple Sclerosis Society

(In the listings below, telephone numbers have symbols V for voice and TDD for tele-communication device for the deaf where organizations have published this information.)

Association of Driver Educators for the Disabled
c/o ADED Secretariat
33736 La Crosse
Westland, MI 48185
(602) 435-9704

Provides information about training and evaluation facilities for driver education for individuals with disabilities.

Medical Rehabilitation Research and Training Center for Multiple Sclerosis
Albert Einstein College of Medicine, Yeshiva University
1300 Morris Park Avenue
New York, NY 10461
(212) 430-2682

This federally funded research and training center performs clinical, behavioral, and biomedical research and offers acute medical and/or surgical care, inpatient rehabilitation, and treatment by a multidisciplinary team.

National Institute of Neurological Disorders and Stroke (NINDS)
National Institutes of Health
Building 31, Room 8A06
Bethesda, MD 20205
(301) 496-5752

A federal agency which conducts basic and clinical research on the causes and treatment of multiple sclerosis.

National Multiple Sclerosis Society
205 East 42nd Street
New York, NY 10017-5706
(800) 624-8236   (212) 986-3240

Provides professional and public education; information and referral; and supports research. Offers counseling services, advocacy, discount prescription and health care products program, and assistance in obtaining adaptive equipment. Local affiliates. Publishes quarterly newsletter, "Inside MS," available in print and on audiocassette. Membership of $20.00 includes newsletter. Individuals with multiple sclerosis may receive a courtesy membership if they are unable to pay.

Facts and Issues
National Multiple Sclerosis Society
205 East 42nd Street
New York, NY 10017-5706

A series of short reports on subjects such as vision loss, pain, pregnancy, and other issues of concern to individuals with multiple sclerosis. Single copy, free.

The Handicapped Driver's Mobility Guide
American Automobile Association
Traffic Safety Department
Handicapped Driver Research
1000 AAA Drive
Heathrow, FL 32746
(407) 444-7963

Provides information about adaptive equipment for automobiles, recreational vehicle and motor home accessories, driver training, service organizations, and publications for drivers with disabilities. Includes U.S., Canadian, and European resources. $3.00; free to AAA members through local divisions.

Living with Low Vision: A Resource Guide for People with Sight Loss
Resources for Rehabilitation
33 Bedford Street, Suite 19A
Lexington, MA 02173
(617) 862-6455

Directs individuals who have experienced vision loss to services, products, and publications that enables them to keep reading, working, and enjoying life. Large print. $35.00 plus $5.00 shipping and handling.

Mastering Multiple Sclerosis
by John K. Wolf
Academy Press, Rutland, VT 05701-0757

Describes the medical aspects of multiple sclerosis and how to manage its symptoms. U.S., $22.95; Canada, $30.45

Moving with Multiple Sclerosis: An Exercise Manual for People with Multiple Sclerosis
by Iris Kimberg
National Multiple Sclerosis Society
205 East 42nd Street
New York, NY 10017-5706
(800) 624-8236   (212) 986-3240

Describes four types of exercises designed to relieve some multiple sclerosis symptoms. Includes passive range of motion and stretching, active and active restrictive, coordination and balance, and exercises to reduce spasticity. Numerous illustrations guide the individual and helper through each exercise sequence. Single copy, free.

MS Quarterly Report
Demos Publications
156 Fifth Avenue, Suite 1018
New York, NY 10010

Describes current basic and clinical research and findings.   U.S. and Canada, $15.00

Multiple Sclerosis: A Guide for Patients and Their Families
by Labe C. Scheinberg (ed.)
Raven Press, New York, NY

Written by physicians, nurses, an occupational therapist, social worker, rehabilitation counselor, and others, this book provides basic information on the causes and course of multiple sclerosis, vocational choices, disability benefits, sexuality, and community resources. Softcover, $15.00; hardcover, $24.50

Multiple Sclerosis Fact Book
by Richard Lechtenberg
FA Davis Company, Philadelphia, PA

Written for the lay person, this book describes up-to-date diagnostic tests and therapies and provides practical ideas for coping with multiple sclerosis. $18.95

PLAINTALK: A Booklet About Multiple Sclerosis For Family Members
by Sarah L. Minden and Debra Frankel
National Multiple Sclerosis Society
205 East 42nd Street
New York, NY 10017-5706
(800) 624-8236   (212) 986-3240

Simulates a support group meeting for families of individuals with multiple sclerosis. Discusses diagnosis, everyday living, talking with children, and the well parent. Single copy, free.

Providing Services for People with Vision Loss
by Susan L. Greenblatt (ed.)
Resources for Rehabilitation
33 Bedford Street, Suite 19A
Lexington, MA 02173
(617) 862-6455

Discusses how health and rehabilitation professionals can work together to provide coordinated care for individuals who have experienced vision loss. Also available on cassette. $19.95 plus $3.00 shipping and handling.

Rehabilitation Resource Manual: VISION
Resources for Rehabilitation
33 Bedford Street, Suite 19A
Lexington, MA 02173
(617) 862-6455

Desk reference which helps health care professionals to make effective referrals for patients with vision loss. Provides information on understanding responses to vision loss and describes optical and nonoptical aids. Hundreds of nationwide referral sources. Chapters on services and products for special population groups and by eye conditions and diseases. $39.95 plus $5.00 shipping and handling.

Sexuality & Multiple Sclerosis
by Michael Barrett
National Multiple Sclerosis Society
205 East 42nd Street
New York, NY 10017-5706
(800) 624-8236   (212) 986-3240

Written for individuals with multiple sclerosis and their partners, this publication discusses the sexual implications of multiple sclerosis, interpersonal relationships, self-image, and self-esteem. Single copy, free.

Symptom Management in Multiple Sclerosis
by Randall T. Shapiro
Demos Publications
156 Fifth Avenue, Suite 1018
New York, NY 10010

A multidisciplinary guide for health care professionals and individuals with multiple sclerosis which suggests management strategies for treating multiple sclerosis and minimizing and controlling its symptoms. Softcover, $10.95; hardcover, $17.95

Talking Books and Multiple Sclerosis
National Library Service for the Blind and Physically Handicapped (NLS)
1291 Taylor Street, NW
Washington, DC 20542
(800) 424-8567

This brochure describes a free program which provides books and magazines recorded on discs and cassettes for individuals with multiple sclerosis. Application forms are available from the NLS, public libraries, or local affiliates of the National Multiple Sclerosis Society. A health professional must certify that the individual is unable to hold a book or turn pages; has blurred or double vision; extreme weakness or excessive fatigue; or other physical limitations which prevent the individual from reading standard print.

Understanding Bladder Dysfunction in Multiple Sclerosis
by Nancy J. Holland and Michele G. Madonna
National Multiple Sclerosis Society
205 East 42nd Street
New York, NY 10017-5706
(800) 624-8236   (212) 986-3240

Describes how multiple sclerosis affects the urinary system; how to control symptoms; and how to manage bladder dysfunction. Single copy, free.

Understanding Multiple Sclerosis
by Robert Shuman and Janice Schwartz
MacMillan Publishing Company, Riverside, NJ

Two psychologists discuss the role of the family with a member who has multiple sclerosis. Includes chapters on adolescents with multiple sclerosis, employment, and research. Uses real life experiences to suggest coping strategies and adaptations. $19.95 plus $1.50 shipping and handling.

SPINAL CORD INJURY

The spinal cord is responsible for transmitting the brain's electrical impulses that control other organs of the body. Therefore, when the spinal cord is injured, there are effects on many of the body's systems, requiring modifications of many activities of everyday living and of the home and workplace environment.

Tumors and diseases such as *poliomyelitis*, *arthritis*, *spina bifida*, and *multiple sclerosis* may cause spinal cord injuries; however, spinal cord injury occurs most frequently as a result of *accidents*. Young males who have been in an automobile accident or a sports accident experience the greatest proportion of spinal cord injuries. Because it is often the case that individuals with spinal cord injury were extremely physically active prior to their injury, the effects of the injury may seem overwhelming to them at first. However, rehabilitation opportunities and the development of a wide variety of special assistive devices have enabled thousands of individuals with spinal cord injury to live productive lives and to continue to participate in many recreational activities, albeit in modified forms.

Studies of patients admitted to regional spinal cord injury centers, which represent admissions of 10% of all individuals with spinal cord injury, have yielded estimates of the incidence of spinal cord injuries and demographic breakdowns (Young et al: 1982). The annual incidence of accidents that cause spinal cord injury where the injured individual survives is between 30 and 35 per million population (approximately eight to ten thousand per year). The average age at onset is 28.7 years, and 82% of individuals with spinal cord injury are males. Automobile accidents are the most common cause of spinal cord injuries. Sports accidents, in particular diving accidents, are a major cause of spinal cord injury among the younger population, while falls are a major cause among the older population.

It has been estimated that there are about 200,000 living Americans who have experienced spinal cord injury, the majority of whom were injured during or after World War II. Prior to World War II and the development of penicillin and of sulfa drugs that prevented death from urinary tract infections, it was unusual for those who had a spinal cord injury to survive (DeVivo et al.: 1987). Today, due to the development of these drugs and improved emergency medical care at the scene of accidents, the vast majority of individuals with spinal cord injury live for many years.

THE SPINAL CORD

The spine has 33 bony, hollow, interlocking vertebrae including seven cervical or neck vertebrae, 12 thoracic or high back vertebrae, five lumbar or low back vertebrae, five sacral vertebrae near the base of the spine, and four coccygeal vertebrae fused to form the coccyx.

The spinal cord, consisting of a narrow bundle of nerve cells and fibers, runs from the base of the brain through the hollow structure of the vertebrae. The brain's communication with the rest of the body is carried out through these nerve fibers.

Paralysis, the loss or impairment of motor function, occurs below the site of the injury or fracture. Not all injuries are complete, meaning that sometimes the individual may retain some sensation or movement below the site of the injury. Paraplegia, or paralysis of the legs and often the lower part of the body, occurs when the spinal cord is injured at the thoracic, lumbar, or sacral level of the spine. When injuries are complete, individuals also lose their sense of touch, pain, and temperature in the affected region.

Quadriplegia (or tetraplegia) is paralysis of all four limbs and the part of the body beneath the site of the spinal cord injury. Quadriplegia occurs when the injury to the spinal cord is at the level of the cervical vertebrae or the neck region. The lower the lesion within the cervical area, the greater amount of function that remains. Some individuals with cervical spinal cord injuries retain some function of the shoulders, biceps, upper arms, and the wrists. In general, the higher the site of the injury, the less function the individual retains. Those individuals whose injuries are complete and at the chin level require respirators in order to breathe. These individuals require assistance with their everyday activities, although the use of mouthsticks and sip-and-puff mechanisms enables them to operate wheelchairs, computers, and other devices (Trieschmann: 1988).

According to Young and his associates (1982), there is a higher prevalence of quadriplegia (53%) than paraplegia (47%), but the injuries are more likely to be complete for paraplegics (60%) than for quadriplegics (52%).

TREATMENT AND COMPLICATIONS OF SPINAL CORD INJURY

Acute medical care following an accident that has caused spinal cord injury includes x-rays, possible treatment for shock, and immobilization of the patient. Patients are often placed in a Stryker frame, which is used to immobilize the spine and prevent further injury. A catheter to control bladder function is inserted and urine output is monitored. In some cases, surgery may be performed to stabilize or fuse the spine, free nerve roots, or remove bony fragments. Immediately following the injury, swelling and bruising near the site of the fracture may be present, preventing the determination of the extent of neurological damage (Trieschmann: 1988). Patients are positioned and turned frequently in an effort to prevent pressure sores (see below). Other injuries that often accompany spinal cord injury, such as fractures and lung injuries, must also be treated. Pain may also be a major problem in the first weeks following injury.

Although treatments have been developed for many of the complications of spinal cord injury, it is still necessary to constantly be aware of the development of these complications and to take measures to prevent them. *Pressure sores* or *decubitus ulcers* are lesions on the skin that usually occur over a bony surface and result from lack of motion. Because the individual may have no sensation at the site where the sores begin to develop, they may become deep before they are discovered. In an effort to prevent pressure sores, individuals who are confined to bed immediately following the injury should be moved frequently and great attention should be paid to cleansing the skin regularly. Special flotation pads and sheepskins are sometimes used to relieve pressure and distribute body weight. Because of their restricted mobility, individuals with spinal cord injury must take precautions to prevent pressure sores for the rest of their lives.

Despite the loss of sensation to temperature and touch below the site of the lesion, *pain* and unusual sensations may be a problem for people with spinal cord injury. According to Trieschmann (1988), until recently it was assumed that pain was not a problem, and little attention was paid to the subject. However, Trieschmann states that many individuals experience a tingling or pins and needles sensation as well as other types of pain, such as shooting or burning sensations.

Transcutaneous electric nerve stimulation (TENS) is a treatment method in which low level electric impulses are delivered to nerve endings under the skin near the source of pain. It is not known why TENS should be effective in relieving pain or if it is really effective. Research is currently underway to gain a better understanding of the way in which this procedure works.

Loss of bladder and bowel control is another complication of spinal cord injury. A recent study (Kuhlemeier et al.: 1985) concluded that patients with spinal cord injury are likely to maintain good renal output ten years after injury. Those individuals who have indwelling catheters are prone to develop bladder infections. When the extent of nerve damage permits, it is preferable to have the individual learn how to control his or her bladder through an individualized training program. Similarly, programs for bowel control enable the individual to empty the bowel on a regular schedule, thereby avoiding gastrointestinal complications such as distention and impaction. Attention to diet and the use of rectal suppositories may also contribute to control of bowel movements.

Spasticity (involuntary jerky motions) is common in individuals with spinal cord injury. These spasms are caused by random stimulation of the nerves leading to the muscles. Severe spasms may interfere with some activity and in some cases may be strong enough to throw the individual from the bed or chair.

Sexual function may be affected in both men and women, although the effects are greater for men. Women will resume menstruating and may conceive and bear children. Because of the loss of motor function, a man's ability to have an erection may be impaired. As with all other effects of spinal cord injury, the extent of the impairment is determined by the level and completeness of the injury. Rehabilitation programs for people with spinal cord injury include counseling in the area of sexual functioning.

As more individuals with spinal cord injuries survive longer, they are also experiencing the normal physiological processes that accompany aging. There is little information on how these processes affect people with spinal cord injury who have been disabled for many years. However, preliminary indications are that physiological changes associated with aging have a greater impact on people with spinal cord injury. Menter (1990) calls this phase "decline," noting that there is a decrease in muscle strength, range of motion, and respiratory and cardiovascular capacity and an increase in the breakdown of the skin.

PSYCHOLOGICAL ASPECTS OF SPINAL CORD INJURY

Individuals who experience spinal cord injury as a result of an accident have had no preparation for life as an individual with a disability. In an instant, they have changed from able-bodied individuals into individuals with severe physical limitations. The suddenness with which this change takes place and the wide ranging effects are likely to cause great anguish to the individuals as well as to their families and friends. The more severe the disability, the greater the loss of independence. For many individuals, these circumstances result in a loss of self-esteem and fear of re-entering the larger community. It is essential that individuals with spinal cord injury receive help with their emotional adjustment, either in the form of individual or group counseling from professionals or through self-help groups and role models of individuals who have adjusted successfully to spinal cord injury.

Indeed, survival itself has found to be positively related to good emotional adjustment following spinal cord injury. Krause and Crewe (1987) compared survivors of spinal cord injury and those who had died several years after their injury on a number of variables that measured adjustment. Those who were better adjusted in terms of vocational and social activity were more likely to survive regardless of their age. Krause and Crewe suggest that the frequent neglect of counseling in social skills and sexual functioning during the rehabilitation process contributes to poor adjustment.

Some individuals may never lose the anger or guilt they feel about the circumstances surrounding the accident that caused the injury. In the period immediately following the accident, they may feel overpowered by the many professionals who have begun to make major decisions for them. In many cases, the accidents that caused spinal cord injury involved the use of alcohol while driving. These factors, combined with inadequate counseling and the inability to cope with the effects of the injury, may cause some individuals to abuse alcohol or other drugs. Bozzacco (1990) suggests that all patients in rehabilitation units be assessed for their vulnerability to alcohol and drug abuse. She further suggests that patients become part of the decision-making process for their own treatment and rehabilitation plans as soon as possible and that alcohol and drug treatment programs be an integral part of rehabilitation.

Because most of the individuals who experience spinal cord injury are males, women who have spinal cord injuries may feel isolated and without accessible peers or role models. They may need counseling about the physical aspects of becoming pregnant; about handling

164

the responsibilities of motherhood; and other physical and emotional issues that affect women.

The need to modify the activities of everyday living as well as the physical environment; the impairment of sexual function; and the financial aspects of living with spinal cord injury may place a great strain on marital and family relationships. In cases where attendant care is necessary, the spouse often becomes a caretaker by default when financial resources do not permit hiring an attendant. In these instances, it is not uncommon for the able-bodied spouse and offspring to feel both overburdened and guilty. Social workers should work with the family to arrange for respite care, financial assistance, and other services that can remediate the situation.

According to Young and his associates (1982), over half (54%) of all individuals with spinal cord injury were single when their injury occurred; these individuals may benefit from counseling in order develop satisfactory relationships and marriage.

WHERE TO FIND SERVICES

The federal government has sponsored the "Model System of Spinal Cord Injury Care" in order to provide coordinated comprehensive care and to conduct research related to spinal cord injury. Administered by the National Institute on Disability and Rehabilitation Research (NIDRR) within the United States Department of Education, this model system encompasses treatment centers throughout the country that participate in research and data collection efforts. According to J. Paul Thomas (1990), who administers this program at NIDRR, the major components of the model system include early access to care through rapid, effective transportation; an acute level one traumatology setting; a comprehensive acute rehabilitation program; psychosocial and vocational services that begin in the hospital and continue through discharge; and follow-up to ascertain that medical and psychosocial needs are met once patients have re-entered the community,.

Another federal system that offers special treatment for individuals with spinal cord injury is the United States Department of Veteran Affairs (VA). Spinal cord units are located at a number of VA Medical Centers across the country. The National Institutes of Health also funds model research and treatment centers at several facilities.

Many rehabilitation hospitals have spinal cord injury units. The advantage of obtaining treatment in these settings is that other patients serve as role models. Some acute care hospitals also have rehabilitation units, and outpatient rehabilitation facilities offer services to people with spinal cord injury. Many long term care facilities provide services to people with spinal cord injury. The Commission on Accreditation of Rehabilitation Facilities (CARF) provides accreditation for these facilities (see "ORGANIZATIONS" section below). Independent living centers offer services and referrals to people with spinal cord injury.

165

PROFESSIONAL SERVICE PROVIDERS

In most cases, the physician in charge serves as the case manager or coordinator for the person with spinal cord injury. The physician in charge may be a *physiatrist* (a specialist trained in rehabilitation medicine); an *orthopedist* (a specialist in treatment of the skeletal system); or a *neurologist* or *neurosurgeon* (a specialist in disorders of the nervous system). All of these physicians receive training in treatment of spinal cord injury. Also on the multidisciplinary team are *urologists*, who specialize in treatment of kidneys, the bladder, the ureter, and the urethra.

Rehabilitation nurses receive special training available at schools throughout the country and may receive certification in this specialty after working two years in a rehabilitation setting (Livingston: 1991). They work closely with the physicians and in some instances may serve as case managers. In in-patient settings, rehabilitation nurses work with other health care and rehabilitation professionals to develop and implement medical and rehabilitation plans for patients. They may act as consultants in planning for the patient's discharge and may evaluate the patient's home to ensure that appropriate environmental modifications have been made. They are often the professionals in charge of following up on the patient's needs after discharge from the rehabilitation unit.

Physical therapists help the person with spinal cord injury with an exercise program designed to maintain and strengthen residual motor function. They also teach the patient transfer skills to and from the bed and how to use wheelchairs and orthotic devices such as canes, braces, and walkers. They develop exercise programs to help individuals who are able to use crutches to build up muscles in their arms and shoulders.

Occupational therapists teach individuals with spinal cord injury how to re-learn the activities of daily living. Included are eating, dressing, grooming, and possibly the use of "high tech" aids that enable the person with spinal cord injury to have increased independence.

Orthotists specialize in the design of braces and other devices that help with mobility, support, and prevention of further injury. They also fit the devices and instruct the patient in their use. *Rehabilitation engineers* specialize in the design of devices that enable people with disabilities to function at their maximum level of independence. Their research includes the development of robotic devices and other computer driven devices that serve as substitutes for the function that was lost as a result of injury or disease. In some instances, they may consult on individual cases to adapt wheelchairs or other devices to the specific needs of the patient.

Psychologists provide individual or group counseling to people with spinal cord injury and to their family members. They may provide special help in the area of sexual functioning for people with spinal cord injury. *Social workers* help to make the arrangements that enable individuals to return to the community. They also ensure that individuals with spinal cord injury receive the financial assistance that they are entitled to. Social workers may also be involved in counseling for individuals and their families.

166

Vocational rehabilitation counselors help individuals with spinal cord injury develop a plan that will enable them to continue functioning and working. Many individuals with spinal cord injury will need assistance in returning to their previous position or retraining to obtain a different type of position. Vocational rehabilitation counselors help make the contacts and placements necessary to attain these goals.

Employment after spinal cord injury is more likely for people who have higher education and who work in office jobs that do not require physical effort. Individuals who were employed in office or clerical work prior to their spinal cord injury are most likely to be able to perform the same type of work, with or without modifications in the office environment. Individuals whose work involved physical skills will in most instances need to be trained to carry out the requirements of more sedentary occupations (For a more detailed discussion of this topic, see Meeting the Needs of Employees with Disabilities described in "PUBLICATIONS AND TAPES" section below).

MODIFICATIONS IN EVERYDAY LIVING

Most individuals with spinal cord injury use wheelchairs for mobility. A wide variety of wheelchairs designed for different purposes and different types of impairments are available. Individuals whose injury prohibits them from using manually operated wheelchairs may use battery operated wheelchairs. Sip-and-puff controls, tubes that respond to changes in pressure caused by inhaling and exhaling, enable people with more severe impairments to control the movement of their wheelchairs. Wheelchairs are prescribed by physicians and must accommodate the individual's body size, disability, and functional criteria.

Individuals whose injury has resulted in paraplegia sometimes use braces as an alternative to wheelchairs. One recent study (Heinemann et al.: 1987) found that only about a quarter of those individuals who had braces continued to use them, while the remainder preferred using wheelchairs. Those who continued to use braces were less likely to have complete lesions than those who stopped using braces. Those who stopped using braces said that they preferred wheelchairs because they were safer, required less energy, and were less likely to fail.

Modification of the home environment requires the installation of ramps; wide doorways with doors that open easily; the removal of thresholds between rooms; and lifts for getting from one level of the home to the other. The kitchen should have accessible appliances, shelves and working space, and easy to use knobs and pulls. The bathroom should be large enough to accommodate a wheelchair; the sink must be at an accessible level; showers should be the roll-in variety with grab bars; and toilets should have grab bars.

Many paraplegics learn to drive with special hand controls, locks, steering mechanisms, and wheelchair lifts. Major automobile manufacturers offer special programs to purchase adapted vehicles with special controls and wheelchair lifts. Parking must be arranged so that there is enough space for entering and exiting the vehicle.

Special feeding devices are available for quadriplegics who do not have the use of their upper limbs. Devices may be installed that move people around a room. Use of these specialized devices increases the independence of quadriplegics. However, quadriplegics do need attendant care to help them carry out their everyday activities. Hiring an attendant can be very expensive, but it is usually preferable to having a family member provide all of the care a quadriplegic needs. Individuals who are eligible for Medicaid or Supplemental Security Income may also be eligible for financial benefits to cover the costs of attendant care.

References

Bozzacco, Victoria
1990 "Vulnerability and Alcohol and Substance Abuse in Spinal Cord Injury" Rehabilitation Nursing 15(Mar.-Apr.):2:70-72

DeVivo, Michael J., Paula L. Kartus, Samuel L. Stover, Richard D. Rutt, and Philip R. Fine
1987 "Seven-Year Survival Following Spinal Cord Injury" Archives of Neurology 44(August):872-875

Heinemann, Allen W., Renee Magiera-Planey, Chrisann Schiro-Geist, and Gloria Gimines
1987 "Mobility for Persons with Spinal Cord Injury: An Evaluation of Two Systems" Archives of Physical Medicine and Rehabilitation 68(February):90-93

Krause, James S. and Nancy M. Crewe
1987 "Prediction of Long-Term Survival of Persons with Spinal Cord Injury: An 11-Year Prospective Study" Rehabilitation Psychology 32:4:205-213

Kuhlemeier, K. V., L.K. Lloyd, and S. L. Stover
1985 "Urological Neurology and Urodynamics" Journal of Urology 134(September):510-513

Livingston, Carolyn
1991 "Opportunities in Rehabilitation Nursing" American Journal of Nursing 91 (Feb.):2:90-95

Menter, Robert R.
1990 "Aging and Spinal Cord Injury: Implications for Existing Model Systems and Future Federal, State, and Local Health Care Policy" pp. 72-80 in David F. Apple and Lesley M. Hudson (eds.) Spinal Cord Injury: The Model Atlanta, GA: Spinal Cord Injury Care System, Sheperd Center for the Treatment of Spinal Injuries

Thomas, J. Paul
1990 "Definition of the Model System of Spinal Cord Injury Care" pp. 7-9 in David F. Apple and Lesley M. Hudson (eds.) <u>Spinal Cord Injury: The Model</u> Atlanta, GA: Spinal Cord Injury Care System, Sheperd Center for the Treatment of Spinal Injuries

Trieschmann, Roberta B.
1988 <u>Spinal Cord Injuries: Psychological, Social and Vocational Rehabilitation</u> New York: Demos

Young, John S., Peter E. Burns, A.M. Bowen, and Roberta McCutchen
1982 <u>Spinal Cord Injury Statistics</u> Phoenix, AZ: Good Samaritan Medical Center

(In the listings below, telephone numbers have symbols V for voice and TDD for tele-communication device for the deaf where organizations have published this information.)

Accent on Living
PO Box 700
Bloomington, IL 61702
(309) 378-2961

A database of assistive devices and how-to information. Publishes "Accent on Living," a quarterly magazine, $8.00 per year, and "Accent on Living Buyers' Guide," $10.95

American Association of Spinal Cord Injury Nursing (AASCIN)
75-20 Astoria Boulevard
Jackson Heights, NY 11370-1178
(718) 803-3782

A professional membership organization that encourages and improves nursing care of individuals with spinal cord injuries and sponsors research. Publishes "SCI Nursing," quarterly. Membership, $25.00

American Paralysis Association (APA)
500 Morris Avenue
Springfield, NJ 07081
(800) 225-0292   (201) 379-2690
Hotline (800) 526-3456   In MD, (800) 638-1733

Supports research to find a cure for paralysis caused by central nervous system disorders and injuries. Publishes "Walking Tomorrow," a newsletter about the organization's activities, and "Progress in Research," a newsletter about spinal cord injury research. Various levels of membership begin at $50.00; subsidized membership available. Also sponsors 24 hour APA Spinal Cord Injury Hotline to answer questions, solve individual problems, and make referrals to professional service providers and peers with spinal cord injuries.

American Paraplegia Society
75-20 Astoria Boulevard
Jackson Heights, NY 11370
(718) 803-3782

A professional membership organization for physicians, scientists, and allied health care professionals. Holds an annual meeting for the presentation of scientific research related to spinal cord injury. Publishes a quarterly journal, "Journal of the American Paraplegia Society," included with membership fee. Membership, $25.00

American Spinal Injury Association (ASIA)
250 East Superior, Room 619
Chicago, IL 60611
(312) 908-3425

A professional membership organization for physicians dedicated to improving the care of patients with spinal cord injury through research, education, and development of regional spinal cord injury care systems. Holds an annual meeting with presentation of scientific papers. Membership, $125.00

Association of Driver Educators for the Disabled
c/o ADED Secretariat
33736 La Crosse
Westland, MI 48185
(602) 435-9704

Provides information about training and evaluation facilities for driver education for individuals with disabilities.

Commission on Accreditation of Rehabilitation Facilities (CARF)
101 North Wilmot Road, Suite 500
Tucson, AZ 85711
(602) 748-1212 (V/TDD)

Conducts site evaluations and accredits organizations that provide rehabilitation.

Functional Electrical Stimulation Information Center
Walker Industrial Rehabilitation Center
10524 Euclid Avenue
Cleveland, OH 44106
(800) 666-2353   (216) 231-3257

A federally funded information and referral clearinghouse affiliated with the Rehabilitation Engineering Center at Case Western Reserve University. Functional electrical stimulation (FES) is an experimental method that uses electrical stimulation to evoke skeletal muscle responses in areas that do not function normally because injury or disease has cut off the pathway for central nervous system communication from the brain. In addition to providing information to consumers and medical professionals about FES, the center develops and evaluates services and products related to FES. Operates an electronic bulletin board; publishes quarterly newsletter, "FES Update," free.

Help for Incontinent People (HIP)
PO Box 544
Union, SC 29379
(803) 579-7902

An information clearinghouse for consumers, family members, and medical professionals. Will answer individual questions if self-addressed stamped envelope is enclosed with letter. Publishes a series of fact sheets; a "Resource Guide of Continence Products and Services," U.S., $10.00; Canada, $11.00; and quarterly newsletter, "The HIP Report," $5.00.

Medical Rehabilitation Research and Training Center in Prevention and Treatment of Secondary Complications of Spinal Cord Injury
Spain Rehabilitation Center
1717 Sixth Avenue South
University of Alabama at Birmingham
Birmingham, AL 35233
(205) 934-3283

A federally funded center that conducts research and holds educational conferences for people with spinal cord injury and their families, six times a year. Also holds training programs for professionals. Publishes a free quarterly newsletter for consumers, "Pushin' On" and an annual "Research Update." The National Spinal Cord Injury Statistical Center collects data from spinal cord injury centers throughout the country. Produces a variety of audio-visual materials and books for professional care providers. A list of articles documenting some of the center's research findings is also available.

National Association of Rehabilitation Facilities (NARF)
PO Box 17675
Washington DC 20041
(703) 648-9300

A national membership organization of individuals and institutions that provide rehabilitation services. Provides seminars, holds an annual meeting, and publishes a series of newsletters.

National Coordinating Council on Spinal Cord Injury (NCCSCI)
801 18th Street, NW
Washington DC 20006
(800) 424-8200   (202) 872-1300

A membership organization for agencies and individuals. Fosters communication among members of the spinal cord injury community and the general public; supports research; and works for the integration of individuals with spinal cord injury into the general community. Publishes a bimonthly newsletter, "Dialogue." Membership, associate $35.00; sponsor $1,000.00; patron $5,000.00.

172

National Institute of Neurological Disorders and Stroke (NINDS)
Information Office
Building 31, Room 8A06
9000 Rockville Pike
Bethesda, MD 20892
(301) 496-5752

Sponsors basic and clinical research to understand, prevent, and cure paralysis. Supports a national program of Spinal Cord Injury Research Centers located at Yale University in New Haven, CT; Ohio State University in Columbus, OH; Medical University of South Carolina in Charleston, SC; and New York University in New York City.

National Institute on Disability and Rehabilitation Research (NIDRR)
U.S. Department of Education
400 Maryland Avenue, SW
Washington DC 20202
(202) 732-1207   (202) 732-1198 (TDD)

A federal agency that supports research into various aspects of disability and rehabilitation, including demographic analyses, social science research, and the development of assistive devices. Supports a nationwide system of model spinal cord injury centers.

National Spinal Cord Injury Association (NSCIA)
800 West Cummings Park, Suite 2000
Woburn, MA 01801
(800) 962-9629   (617) 935-2722

A membership organization with chapters throughout the United States. Disseminates information to people with spinal cord injuries and to their families; provides counseling; and advocates for the removal of barriers to independent living. Participates in the development of standards of care for regional spinal cord injury care. Holds annual meeting and educational seminars. Membership includes quarterly magazine, "Spinal Cord Injury Life," fact sheets, and discounts on other publications. Membership, $25.00 for individual with disability or family member; $35.00 professional; $100.00 organizational.

Paralyzed Veterans of America (PVA)
801 18th Street NW
Washington, DC 20006
(800) 424-8200   (202) 416-7619

A membership organization for veterans with spinal cord injury. Advocates and lobbies for the rights of paralyzed veterans and sponsors research. Publishes "Paraplegia News" and "Sports-n-Spokes" (see "PUBLICATIONS AND TAPES" section below). Membership fees are set by state chapters. To locate the chapter nearest you, phone the national office.

The PVA Spinal Cord Injury Education and Training Foundation accepts applications to fund continuing education; post-professional specialty training; and patient/client and family education. The PVA Spinal Cord Research Foundation accepts applications to fund basic and clinical research; the design of assistive devices; and conferences that foster interaction among scientists and health care providers.

Rehabilitation R & D Center
VA Medical Center
3801 Miranda Avenue/ 153
Palo Alto, CA 94304-1200

Develops prosthetics, robots, adaptations for wheelchairs, and other assistive devices. Publishes, "OnCenter," a newsletter that discusses recent developments at the center, free.

Rehabilitation Research and Training Center for Treatment of Secondary Complications of Spinal Cord Injury
Department of Rehabilitation Medicine
Northwestern University
345 East Superior Street
Chicago, IL 60611
(312) 908-6017

A federally funded center that conducts research and training on the prevention and treatment of secondary complications of spinal cord injury.

Rehabilitation Research and Training Center in Community-Oriented Services for Persons with Spinal Cord Injury
Department of Rehabilitation Medicine
Baylor College of Medicine
One Baylor Plaza
Houston, TX 77030
(713) 799-7011

A federally funded center that conducts research and training on the health needs, psychological adjustment, and community integration of individuals with spinal cord injury.

Simon Foundation
PO Box 815
Wilmette, IL 60091
(708) 864-3913

Provides information and assistance to people who are incontinent. Publishes a monthly newsletter, "The Informer." Organizes self-help groups. (See "PUBLICATIONS AND TAPES" section below.)

<u>VA Office of Technology Transfer</u>
Prosthetics R&D Center
103 South Gay Street
Baltimore, MD 21202
(301) 962-1800

Sponsors rehabilitation research and development of assistive technology. Publishes "Journal of Rehabilitation Research and Development" (see "PUBLICATIONS AND TAPES" section below). The VA Rehabilitation Database includes abstracts of articles in the "Journal of Rehabilitation Research and Development," a section on wheelchairs for adults, adaptive automotive equipment, and information on other assistive devices. The database is available through CompuServe, a subscription computer network. Call Dori Grasso at the number listed above for help or for free introductory time on CompuServe.

<u>Vocational Rehabilitation Services</u>
Veterans Benefits Administration
Department of Veterans Affairs (VA)
810 Vermont Avenue, NW
Washington DC 20420
(202) 233-6496

Provides education and rehabilitation assistance and independent living services to veterans with service related disabilities through offices located in every state as well as regional centers, medical centers, and insurance centers. Medical services are provided at VA Medical Centers, Outpatient Clinics, Domiciliaries, and Nursing Homes.

Aerobics for Paraplegics and
Aerobics for Quadriplegics
National Handicapped Sports/Videotapes
1145 19th Street, NW, Suite 717
Washington DC 20036
(301) 652-7505   (301) 652-0119 (TDD)

In each of these videotapes, a person with the disability demonstrates a specially created exercise routine. Single title, $15.00; both titles $28.00; plus $4.50 shipping and handling.

American Institute on Architects (AIA)
1735 New York Avenue, NW
Washington, DC 20006
(202) 626-7300

Publishes two bibliographies related to disabilities: one of books in AIA Reference Library (number B 100) and one of periodical article citations (number P 131) on barrier-free design. Free for members; nonmembers, $15.00 per bibliography. "Americans with Disabilities Act Information Kit" describes the ADA's effect on the field of architecture; members, $9.95; nonmembers, $16.95.

A Consumer's Guide to Home Adaptation
The Adaptive Environments Center
374 Congress Street, Suite 301
Boston, MA 02210
(617) 695-1225 (V/DD)

A workbook that enables people with mobility impairments to plan the modifications necessary to adapt their homes. Includes descriptions of widening doorways, lowering countertops, etc. $9.50

The First Whole Rehab Catalog
by A. Jay Abrams and Margaret Ann Abrams
Betterway Publications, Inc.
PO Box 219
Crozet, VA 22932
(804) 823-5661

Describes adaptive aids and products for independent living. $16.95

The Handicapped Driver's Mobility Guide
American Automobile Association (AAA)
Traffic Safety Department
Handicapped Driver Research
1000 AAA Drive
Heathrow, FL 32746
(407) 444-7963

Provides information about adaptive equipment for automobiles, recreational vehicle and motor home accessories, driver training, service organizations, and publications for drivers with disabilities. Includes U.S., Canadian, and European resources. Free to AAA members through local divisions; nonmembers, $3.00.

Journal of Rehabilitation Research and Development (JRRD)
Office of Technology Transfer
VA Prosthetics R&D Center
103 South Gay Street
Baltimore, MD 21202

A quarterly publication of scientific and engineering articles related to spinal cord injury, prosthetics and orthotics, sensory aids, and gerontology. Includes abstracts of literature, book reviews, and calendar of events. A special issue on choosing a wheelchair system appeared as Clinical Supplement # 2 to the March, 1990 edition. For sale by U.S. Superintendent of Documents, Government Printing Office, Washington DC 20402

Living with Spinal Cord Injury
by Barry Corbett
Fanlight Productions
47 Halifax Street
Boston, MA 02130
(617) 542-0980

A series of three videotapes produced by an individual who has experienced spinal cord injury himself. "Changes" is about the consequences of spinal cord injury and the process of rehabilitation. "Outside" emphasizes the life-long aspect of rehabilitation for people with spinal cord injury. "Survivors" interviews 23 men and women who have lived at least 24 years with spinal cord injury. May be rented or purchased. Purchase of single 16mm film, $300.00; rental $50.00. Purchase of videotape, $250.00; rental $100.00. Add $9.00 shipping.

Managing Incontinence
Simon Foundation
PO Box 815
Wilmette, IL 60091
(708) 864-3913

Provides medical advice, information on products, interviews with individuals who are incontinent, and advice on sexuality. $11.95

National Resource Directory
National Spinal Cord Injury Association (NSCIA)
800 West Cummings Park, Suite 2000
Woburn, MA 01801
(800) 962-9629   (617) 935-2722

A reference book with information on medical aspects of spinal cord injury, legal rights, independent living, and a bibliography. $20.00 or included with membership in NSCIA (see "ORGANIZATIONS" section above)

Paraplegia News
5201 North 19th Avenue, Suite 111
Phoenix, AZ 85015

A monthly magazine sponsored by the Paralyzed Veterans of America (See "ORGANI-ZATIONS" section above). Features information for paralyzed veterans and civilians, articles about everyday living, new legislation, employment, and research. U.S., $12.00; foreign, $20.00

Resources: A National Directory of Spinal Cord Injury Prevention Programs
Medical Rehabilitation Research and Training Center in Prevention and Treatment of Secondary Complications of Spinal Cord Injury
Spain Rehabilitation Center
1717 Sixth Avenue South
University of Alabama at Birmingham
Birmingham, AL 35233
(205) 934-3283

Describes over 150 spinal cord injury prevention programs throughout the United States. Includes information on popular audio-visual materials and how to start a training program. $9.95

Spinal Cord Injury Home Care Manual
Rehab. Educational Fund
Santa Clara Valley Medical Center
751 South Bascom Avenue
San Jose, CA 95128-2699

Provides people with spinal cord injury, their families, and professionals with information about physical care, independent living, psychosocial issues, attendant care, and supplies. $50.00

<u>Spinal Cord Injury Life</u>
National Spinal Cord Injury Association (NSCIA)
800 West Cummings Park, Suite 2000
Woburn, MA 01801
(800) 962-9629   (617) 935-2722

A quarterly magazine that provides information about the NSCIA, legislation, research, and new products. Available free with membership in the NSCIA or $20.00 for annual subscription.

<u>Spinal Network</u>
by Sam Maddox
PO Box 4162
Boulder, CO 80306
(800) 338-5412   (303) 449-5412

Describes the medical aspects of spinal cord injury and the wide variety of effects on everyday living. Presents numerous biographical accounts of people who have lived with spinal cord injury. Discusses many issues of everyday living, including recreation and sports, travel, legal and financial aspects. $27.95 plus $4.00 shipping "Spinal Network Extra" is a quarterly magazine with updated information and new articles on similar topics. $15.00

<u>Sports 'N Spokes</u>
5201 North 19th Avenue, Suite 111
Phoenix, AZ 85015

A bimonthly magazine that features articles about sports activities for people who use wheelchairs. U.S., $9.00; foreign, $14.00

<u>The Wheelchair Traveler</u>
Accent on Living
PO Box 700
Bloomington, IL 61702
(309) 378-2961

A directory that rates hotels and motels in the United States. $20.00 plus $1.50 shipping

VISUAL IMPAIRMENT AND BLINDNESS

The number of people with visual impairments has increased dramatically in recent years. Two major factors have contributed to the increase in visual impairment. First, advances in technology have enabled very low birth weight babies to survive, often with serious disabilities including visual impairment. Second, the number of older people, who account for a large portion of the population with vision loss, has increased rapidly. It is projected that the older population will continue to grow and that by the year 2030, there will be 35 million Americans age 65 years or older (Fowles: 1988).

Recent data from the U.S. Census Bureau (1986) indicate that nearly 13 million Americans age 15 years or older report having problems reading ordinary newsprint, even with the use of corrective lenses. Because this statistic represents a self-report of visual impairment, it does not provide a standardized measure; nonetheless, it does suggest that visual impairment is one of the major physical disabilities in the United States. Of ten impairments studied by the National Center for Health Statistics (1981), visual impairment had the second highest prevalence rate and the largest rate of increase from 1971 to 1977.

MAJOR TYPES AND CAUSES OF VISUAL IMPAIRMENT AND BLINDNESS

Low vision is the term that is commonly used to refer to visual impairments that leave the individual with some residual vision. Although there are no standard definitions of low vision, professionals usually consider an acuity of 20/70 or worse to be low vision. In the United States, individuals are considered *legally blind* if they have a visual acuity of 20/200 or worse in the better eye with all possible correction (glasses) or a field restriction of 20 degrees diameter or less in the better eye. Most individuals who are legally blind retain some useful vision and should be encouraged to use it to the maximum extent possible. The classification of legal blindness entitles American citizens to tax benefits and to rehabilitation services provided by state governments. Definitions of legal blindness vary in other countries. A relatively small proportion of the population that is visually impaired or blind have only light perception or are totally blind.

Central vision loss and peripheral field loss are two major types of visual impairment. *Central vision* enables people to read and to recognize faces. The retina, which is at the posterior of the eye, acts as the eye's camera. In the center of the retina is the macula, a small area that is responsible for detailed vision. Damage to the macula affects central vision. To compensate for this loss, a person with macular disease may sometimes appear to be looking at another person's face out of the side of his or her eyes.

Individuals use *peripheral vision* for mobility and to see the full scope of the scene they are facing. Diminished peripheral vision is often referred to as tunnel vision. This impairment affects mobility, although the central vision may still be intact. Some progressive diseases, such as glaucoma, begin with loss of peripheral vision but may progress to total loss of vision, including central vision.

The leading causes of visual impairment or blindness are macular degeneration, glaucoma, diabetic retinopathy, and cataract. Other conditions which may lead to vision loss are corneal diseases, retinitis pigmentosa, stroke, retinal detachment, trauma, and tumors. Blindness or vision loss in children may be caused by congenital deficits, hereditary conditions, or diseases such as retinoblastoma, a cancer of the eye.

Macular degeneration describes a variety of diseases that cause the macula to deteriorate. Age-related macular degeneration (AMD) is the most common form of macular degeneration. It occurs most frequently among the population age 50 or older, and it is the leading cause of vision loss among Americans age 65 or older. Central vision is affected, but some useful central vision often remains. Distortion of straight lines or a loss of clarity in the central field of vision are common symptoms of macular degeneration. Laser treatment has been found to temporarily halt the progressive vision loss in some cases of macular degeneration.

In *glaucoma*, elevated intra-ocular pressure may damage the optic disk and cause changes to the peripheral visual field. Glaucoma is often not diagnosed until the late stages of the disease, because symptoms are not present in the early stages. When symptoms do appear, they are in the form of peripheral field defects and blurred vision. Routine ophthalmic examinations are recommended in order to detect asymptomatic diseases such as glaucoma. Medication, in the form of either pills or eye drops, is used to decrease intra-ocular pressure. Treating glaucoma may halt its progression, but sight that has been lost cannot be restored.

A *cataract* is an opacity or clouding of the lens of the eye which causes decreased visual acuity. Blurred vision, reduced contrast sensitivity, reduced color perception, and difficulty with reading and night driving are some of the symptoms of cataracts. When a cataract interferes with an individual's functional vision, it may be removed by surgery. When the cataract is removed, the most common substitute for the lens is an intra-ocular lens (IOL), which is placed in the eye surgically. Contact lenses, for those who have the manual dexterity to use them, or thick glasses are other choices. If the cataract is present with other eye diseases that cause reduced vision, removal of the cataract will not restore normal vision.

The major cause of visual impairment in young adults is *diabetic retinopathy*. Diabetes may cause damage to the small blood vessels in the eye,which in turn fail to nourish the retina adequately. Bleeding may occur inside the eye. Laser therapy is often used to stop the bleeding. Blood from damaged blood vessels in the eye seeps into the vitreous, blocking the passage of light to the retina. A surgical procedure known as a vitrectomy may be used in an attempt to restore vision. The vitreous or gel which fills the eye between the lens and the retina, is replaced with a saline solution. (For more detailed information about vision loss, see Rehabilitation Resource Manual: VISION, described in "PUBLICATIONS AND TAPES" section below under the "Living with Low Vision Series.")

VISUAL IMPAIRMENT AND BLINDNESS IN CHILDREN

A recent study reports an increase in the rates of congenital blindness since 1970 and evidence that there are many more children who are visually impaired or blind being served in schools (Kirchner: 1990). *Retinopathy of prematurity* (formerly known as retrolental fibroplasia) is one cause of the increase in congenital blindness. Retinopathy of prematurity (ROP) describes an eye condition in which there is a growth of abnormal blood vessels and scar tissue in the eyes of some low birth weight premature infants. First observed in the 1940's, this condition was formerly attributed to the use of excessive oxygen in the incubators. Research no longer supports this single cause (Zierler: 1988). Other factors which have been implicated are vitamin A and E deficiencies; low oxygen and high carbon dioxide blood levels; and other metabolic factors (Repka: 1989). Most researchers agree that prematurity itself and low birth weight are primary contributors to retinopathy of prematurity. Long-term complications observed in older children and young adults include retinal detachment and narrow-angle glaucoma (Repka: 1989). Therefore individuals with retinopathy of prematurity should receive regular ophthalmological examinations throughout their lives.

Macular degeneration, described above as a major cause of visual impairment in adults, may also be present in infants, children, and adolescents. The hereditary form of macular degeneration is called "juvenile macular degeneration." Reduced visual acuity is the primary symptom. Although there is no treatment for this condition, glasses and low vision aids enable individuals to function independently.

Other conditions which cause vision loss or blindness in children are *congenital cataracts*, *congenital glaucoma*, *aniridia* (a partial or complete absence of the iris), and *albinism*. Some of these conditions may lead to further visual loss as children grow older.

VISUAL IMPAIRMENT AND BLINDNESS IN ELDERS

Visual impairment increases elders' awareness of the decline of their physical powers and makes them intimately familiar with the incapacities of old age (Ainlay: 1989, 95). It is difficult for a person to mobilize strengths and compensate for the loss of vision by sharpening the use of other senses when those other senses are also deteriorating and strengths are diminishing (Associated Services for the Blind: 1988).

The individual's personal and social independence is affected, influencing attitudes and emotional status, as well as the ability to adapt to loss. In addition, vision loss is responsible for many of the falls experienced by elders; the misuse of medication when labels cannot be read; and driving accidents (Wright: 1986). (For a more detailed discussion of the ways in which vision loss affects elders and services available to help them, see <u>Resources for Elders with Disabilities</u>, described in "PUBLICATIONS AND TAPES" section below.)

PSYCHOLOGICAL ASPECTS OF VISION LOSS

Vision loss affects all aspects of life. Individuals who have experienced vision loss fear that they will lose their jobs and the ability to support themselves; that they will be unable to take care of themselves; and that they will become the object of pity. Vision loss threatens independence, which in turn diminishes self-esteem. When self-esteem is low, it is often difficult to accept assistance offered by others, including services from professionals.

Individuals with vision loss often need time to adjust psychologically before they are able to begin the rehabilitation process. The amount of time that individuals need before they accept their vision loss and are able to benefit from rehabilitation is a personal matter and may be a matter of days, months, or even years. In many cases, individuals who are slow to accept their prognosis will benefit from speaking to others who have gone through similar experiences or from discussing the situation with a professional counselor.

Progressive vision loss often affects the individual's educational and career plans. An explanation of the likely progression of an individual's eye condition or disease and early referrals for services will facilitate the adjustment process. It will also help individuals make career choices. For example, young people with retinitis pigmentosa or juvenile macular degeneration must be made aware that careers as airplane pilots or surgeons are unrealistic. However, people with these conditions may succeed in a wide variety of demanding professional careers, often with the assistance of adaptive equipment.

Some forms of visual impairment or blindness are hereditary, such as albinism, some retinitis pigmentosa syndromes, congenital cataracts, aniridia, and congenital glaucoma. Parents often feel guilty when their children are diagnosed with a hereditary condition that causes visual impairment or blindness. It is often helpful for parents to attend support groups, where they can talk about their feelings and about methods that their family can use to cope with the child's visual impairment or blindness. Genetic counselors may be able to provide information that will help parents decide whether or not to have more children. Learning about the many services, educational programs, and products that enable individuals who are visually impaired or blind to function independently will help alleviate parents' anxieties about their child's future.

Individuals are often unaware of the causes of visual impairment or blindness or the services provided by health and rehabilitation professionals in the field of vision loss. Individuals with vision loss are an underserved group within the general population, and even more dramatically, in the older population. Not only do elders tend to view loss of vision as an inevitable part of aging and therefore fail to seek support services, but professionals working with elders also tend to have this attitude (Branch et al: 1989). The role of professional service providers may be crucial in determining individual and family responses to the diagnosis of visual impairment or blindness.

An *ophthalmologist* (M.D.) is a physician who specializes in diseases of the eye and systemic diseases that affect the eye's functioning. An *optometrist* (O.D.) is trained to conduct refractions and prescribe corrective lenses. In some states, optometrists are also licensed to administer drugs. An *optician* is trained to make and dispense corrective lenses. All of these practitioners should refer patients for rehabilitation services when medical or surgical treatment and the prescription of corrective lenses do not result in normal visual acuity.

A *low vision specialist* may be an ophthalmologist, optometrist, optician, or other professional who is trained to help individuals with vision loss make use of their remaining vision to the greatest extent possible through the use of optical and nonoptical aids.

A *rehabilitation counselor* serves as a case coordinator for individuals who are visually impaired or blind and require rehabilitation services. The rehabilitation counselor establishes a one-to-one relationship in the initial interview. In succeeding contacts, the rehabilitation counselor and the individual jointly develop an Individual Written Rehabilitation Plan that is appropriate and realistic. Rehabilitation guidelines have been revised to include the role of "homemaker" as a justifiable rehabilitation goal.

A *rehabilitation teacher* provides individualized instruction in activities of daily living. This instruction may include practical adaptations such as large print telephone dials; markers for stoves, thermostats, and medications; and suggestions to increase home safety. The rehabilitation teacher also provides information about community resources and services.

An *orientation and mobility* (O and M) instructor orients the individual to his or her home, the immediate areas outside the home, and teaches safe travel skills using the long white cane.

A *vision teacher* works with the parents of a child who is visually impaired or blind to develop an Individualized Education Plan (IEP) which outlines specific instruction, special equipment, and other services to be provided to the child. Vision teachers may provide instruction in typing, braille, and orientation and mobility, while serving as a resource to classroom teachers on methods of working with the child in a regular classroom.

Other health professionals who may be involved in the care of individuals with visual impairment or blindness are *occupational therapists*, *geriatricians*, *diabetologists*, and mental health professionals such as *psychologists*, *psychiatrists*, and *social workers*.

WHERE TO FIND SERVICES

Services for people who are visually impaired or blind are often offered in ophthalmologists' or optometrists' offices, hospitals, and private or public rehabilitation agencies. These services include the prescription of optical and nonoptical aids which enable individuals to make maximum use of their remaining vision or provide an alternative to visual tasks.

In many states, ophthalmologists and optometrists are required to register individuals who are legally blind with the state agency responsible for serving individuals who are visually impaired or blind, either a "Commission for the Blind" or a division of the state vocational rehabilitation agency. Most public agencies require that clients be legally blind in order to receive services. If individuals do not know if they are legally blind, they should ask an ophthalmologist or optometrist. Some agencies which have the word "blind" in their names serve individuals with varying degrees of visual impairment, including low vision. Many private agencies also serve individuals with vision loss; they are usually listed in the "Social Service Organizations" section of the Yellow Pages or in the "Community Services" section of the white pages of local telephone directories.

Children who are visually impaired or blind are eligible for services mandated by the Individuals with Disabilities Education Act (formerly called the Education of the Handicapped Act) and early intervention programs which are available to all children with disabilities (see Chapter 3, "Children and Youth"). Elders who have experienced vision loss but who are not legally blind may be eligible for services from a state department on aging or elder affairs or an area agency on aging. Veterans with vision loss are eligible for services from VA Medical Centers throughout the country, whether or not their vision loss is service-connected.

ENVIRONMENTAL ADAPTATIONS

The following adaptations are recommended to help people who are visually impaired but who retain some useful vision to function in their homes, schools, and community centers as well as in health and rehabilitation service providers' offices.

Increasing the size of an object projects it on to a larger part of the retina. Using a bold point pen with black ink for writing or large print labels for telephone dials or push-buttons are two simple examples. Large print books or video magnifiers, which enlarge print on a screen, also make reading easier.

Move closer to the object. Individuals may need to sit closer to the television or hold a book or newspaper closer to their eyes. Children in school may need to sit closer to the chalkboard.

Increase the amount of light. Many individuals with vision loss may find that two to three times more light than usual is necessary. Fluorescent lights diffuse evenly and are inexpensive, but they produce less contrast, may flicker, and are harsh. Diffusing filters may solve these problems. The incandescent light found in a standard bulb offers more contrast and can be directed, but it produces shadows and glare. Diffusers and additional lighting spread the light around and reduce shadows. A combination is often the best choice; fluorescent for general lighting, incandescent for near tasks. Sunlight is natural and bright but not easily controlled.

Control glare. Dimmer switches are useful in controlling glare. Sunglasses worn indoors are helpful in controlling the glare from overhead lights. Many individuals find that an amber tint controls glare without sacrificing clarity. A night light is useful when rising in a dark room or walking down a dark hall. It reduces accommodation problems and avoids the need to turn on a bright light. Even individuals who have very little functional vision complain of problems with glare and may benefit from these suggestions.

Change or improve contrast. Color perception is often reduced in individuals who are visually impaired. Light/dark color combinations in wall and hallway colors; painted or carpeted stairs in a color that contrasts with the floor above and below; white or light colored dishes on colored tablecloths; and pouring liquids against light or dark backgrounds are useful strategies to overcome color perception deficits. Painting stripes or placing tape in contrasting colors on the edges of steps and marking stove and thermostat dials with dots of brightly colored glues are other practical adaptations.

The following adaptations are recommended for people who have severe visual impairments or no useful vision. People with less severe visual impairments often utilize these techniques as well.

Use other senses. An individual who becomes visually impaired or blind does not develop a "sixth sense," as is commonly believed. However, individuals learn to use their remaining senses more effectively. Talking calculators, talking watches, and talking clocks provide information aurally; tape recorders are used to take messages; recorded publications played on special tape players provide hours of enjoyment. Items such as canned or frozen foods, spools of thread, or articles of clothing may be marked with tactile labels. Raised large print letters, braille, or special glues which leave a raised "dot" may be used.

Braille uses the sense of touch as an alternative method of reading and writing. Raised dots in various combinations represent the letters of the alphabet, numbers, and punctuation. Most individuals who read and write braille use Grade II braille, which employs the use of contractions, special combinations of letters used in place of an actual word or part of a word. For example, contractions substitute for prepositions such as "with" and "through." Word

186

endings such as "ing" or "ed" use a single symbol, rather than writing each letter of the word ending. Most individuals use a slate and stylus or a braillewriter to produce braille text. The individual using a slate and stylus punches each letter into a cell which accommodates up to six dots (all braille letters, numbers, and contractions, are combinations of one to six dots). Braille is written from right to left so that when the paper is removed from the slate and turned over, the raised dots may be read from left to right. A braillewriter uses six keys, one key for each dot in the braille cell. The user taps various combinations of keys to produce letters, numbers, and punctuation. Braille text may also be produced using a computer and a braille printer.

Most individuals who are congenitally blind use braille as their major reading and writing technique. Blind children should also learn to use a regular typewriter at an early age so that they can communicate in writing with sighted people. Braille literacy has decreased in recent years. The factors that have contributed to this decrease include a decrease in the number of professionals who teach braille; the development and use of low vision aids; and mainstreaming children who are visually impaired or blind into regular classes. Individuals who lose vision as adults are less likely to learn braille, especially those whose vision loss is due to the complications of diabetes. These individuals often lose sensitivity in their fingertips and cannot read braille's raised dots. People of any age who are motivated may learn braille from a rehabilitation teacher or teacher of the visually impaired; through correspondence courses; or in braille classes offered in rehabilitation programs. Some individuals with a diminished sense of touch use "jumbo" braille, written with a slate or braillewriter which produces larger dots. Braille users also use recorded materials and computers with speech or braille output.

Special closed-channel radio receivers are used to provide *radio reading services* to individuals with a print-handicap, either visual or physical (inability to hold a book or turn pages). Newspapers, books, and local information are read in a recording studio and broadcast over a network of radio reading services. Audio description or *Descriptive Video Service* (DVS) makes television programs or theatrical performances accessible to audiences who are visually impaired or blind. A description is provided of the action taking place, the setting, the actors' clothing, and other visual details. Viewers receive DVS through a stereo television, a videocassette recorder which has a Separate Audio Program (SAP) channel, or a stereo television adapter (see "ORGANIZATIONS" section below).

Family members and professionals may find the following guidelines helpful when living or working with individuals who are visually impaired or blind:

> • Always be certain that the individual knows that you are talking
> to him or her. Use a normal speaking voice unless you know that
> the individual has a hearing loss. Always look the individual in the
> eye when speaking.

> • Use sighted guide technique: the person who is visually impaired

or blind holds the arm of the sighted person just above the elbow and follows a few steps behind. (An orientation and mobility instructor or a rehabilitation teacher can provide instruction in this simple technique.)

• Tell the individual when you are entering or leaving the room.

• If in doubt about whether individuals need help, simply ask if they need assistance.

ASSISTIVE DEVICES

There are many useful aids and devices which help individuals who are visually impaired or blind to live independently. One of the simplest aids is the bold pen, available in stationery stores. Other simple writing aids include bold line paper and signature guides.

Banking is easier with large print checks, deposit slips and check registers. A check writing guide fits over a standard check and provides window guides for filling out the check. Some banks offer special services to customers who are visually impaired or blind, including cassette bank statements. Some automated teller machines are accessible through the use of braille labels or step-by-step telephone instructions.

Large print reading materials are very popular with individuals who are visually impaired. In addition to popular fiction works, reference books, cookbooks, bibles, and other religious materials are available in large print. Most public libraries have large print collections. Many publications are recorded on cassette or flexible discs (thin plastic records) by organizations such as the National Library Service for the Blind and Physically Handicapped (NLS) and Recording for the Blind (RFB). Although RFB requires that individuals be legally blind in order to use its services, anyone with a print-handicap is eligible for NLS services (see "ORGANIZATIONS" section below). Full-length and abridged books are available on audiocassette from local bookstores and libraries.

Telephones may be adapted with large print or braille dials or push-button labels. Self-threading needles and large print, cassette, or braille instruction books allow individuals who are visually impaired or blind to continue with sewing and other handcrafts. Large print or braille letters on self-adhesive tape, raised dots, and special glues may be used to label items such as canned goods, medications, and appliances. Recreational items such as playing cards, bingo cards, or crossword puzzle books are available in large print versions. Braille versions of board games such as Scrabble and Monopoly are available. Large print or tactile watches and talking watches, and clocks, thermometers, and blood sugar monitors are additional devices that help individuals manage their everyday activities.

References

Ainlay, Stephen C.
1989 <u>Day Brought Back My Night: Aging and New Vision Loss</u> London and New York: Routledge

Associated Services for the Blind
1988 <u>Volunteers for the Visually Impaired Elderly: A Coordinated Approach to Service Delivery</u> Philadelphia, PA: Associated Services for the Blind

Branch, Lawrence G., Amy Horowitz, and Cheryl Carr
1989 "The Implications for Everyday Life of Incident Self-Reported Visual Decline Among People Over Age 65 Living in the Community" <u>The Gerontologist</u> 29(March):359-365

Fowles, D.
1988 <u>A Profile of Older Americans</u> Washington, D.C.: American Association of Retired People

Kirchner, Corrinne
1990 "Trends in the Prevalence Rates and Numbers of Blind and Visually Impaired Schoolchildren" <u>Journal of Visual Impairment and Blindness</u> 84:9:478-9

Repka, Michael X.
1989 "Update on Retinopathy of Prematurity" <u>Future Reflections</u> 8:3:29-31

U.S. Census Bureau
1986 <u>Disability, Functional Limitation, and Health Insurance Coverage:1984/85</u> Current Population Reports, Series P-70, No. 8, Washington DC: U.S. Government Printing Office

Wright, Irving S.
1987 "Keeping an Eye on the Rest of the Body" <u>Ophthalmology</u> 94(September):1196-1198

Zierler, Sally
1988 "Causes of Retinopathy of Prematurity: An Epidemiologic Perspective" pp. 23-33 in John T. Flynn and Dale L. Phelps (eds.) <u>Retinopathy of Prematurity: Problem and Challenge</u> New York, NY: Alan R. Liss, Inc.

(In the listings below, telephone numbers have symbols V for voice and TDD for tele-communication device for the deaf where organizations have published this information.)

American Council of the Blind (ACB)
1155 15th Street, NW, Suite 702
Washington, DC 20005
(800) 424-8666   (202) 467-5081

National membership organization that provides information and advocates on behalf of individuals who are visually impaired or blind. Has special interest divisions for government employees, students, etc. Makes referrals to local affiliates. Publishes the "Braille Forum," a bimonthly magazine, available in large print, braille, 4-track cassette (playable only on a National Library Service Talking Book Cassette Player), and IBM disk. Shares parenting information between blind/sighted parents of blind/sighted children. Membership, $5.00

American Foundation for the Blind (AFB)
15 West 16th Street
New York, NY 10011
(800) 232-5463   (212) 620-2000

A national information clearinghouse on blindness and vision impairment. "Public Education Materials Catalogue," free.

American Printing House for the Blind (APH)
1839 Frankfort Avenue
PO Box 6085
Louisville, KY 40206-0085
(502) 895-2405

A major resource for educational materials in large print and braille. Manufactures equipment and adaptive aids. Also sells braille children's books at reasonable prices.

Architectural and Transportation Barriers Compliance Board
1111 18th Street, NW, Suite 501
Washington DC 20036-3894
(800) 872-2253 (V/TDD)   (202) 653-7834 (V/TDD)

A federal agency charged with assisting federal personnel and others in setting accessibility standards mandated by federal law. Provides technical assistance, sponsors research, and distributes publications.

Association for the Education and Rehabilitation of the Blind and Visually Impaired (AER)
206 North Washington Street
Alexandria, VA 22314
(703) 548-1884

Membership organization of rehabilitation counselors and teachers, orientation and mobility instructors, special educators, and other professionals with an interest in visual impairment. Publishes newsletter, "AER Report;" holds regional and international meetings; sets standards for certification. Membership fee of $50.00 includes subscription to "RE:view," a quarterly journal.

Association for Macular Diseases
210 East 64th Street
New York, NY 10021
(212) 605-3719

Membership organization which produces newsletter, provides public education, support, and a hot-line for macular degeneration patients. Membership, $20.00

Blind Babies Foundation
50 Oak Street, Suite 102
San Francisco, CA 94102
(415) 863-5464

Provides support, education, referrals, and resources for families with children age birth through five who are visually impaired or blind. PAVII Parents Project Packet, $5.00. Newsletter, "Horizons."

Blind Children's Center
4120 Marathon Street
PO Box 29159
Los Angeles, CA 90029-0159
(800) 222-3566   (213) 664-2153

Offers a free educational correspondence course that answers questions about raising a child who is visually impaired or blind. Telephone consultations also available. Free publications include "Talk to Me I," "Talk to Me II," "Learning to Play: Common Concerns for the Visually Impaired Preschool Child," and "Heart-to-Heart - Parents of Blind and Visually Impaired Children Talk About Their Feelings" (available in Spanish).

Blinded Veterans Association (BVA)
477 H Street, NW
Washington DC 20001
(202) 371-8880

The BVA's field service program helps veterans find rehabilitation, services, and training. The Outreach Employment Program helps veterans find jobs. Publishes the "Bulletin" in large print and on disc.

Canadian National Institute for the Blind (CNIB)
1931 Bayview Avenue
Toronto, Ontario M4G 4C8 Canada
(416) 480-7580

Provides rehabilitation services and counseling to Canadians with any degree of functional vision impairment. Operates resource centres and technology centres and provides special services for seniors, veterans, and people who are deaf-blind. Public information literature available. Contact the National Office for addresses of provincial and local CNIB offices.

Council for Exceptional Children (CEC)
1920 Association Drive
Reston, VA 22091
(703) 620-3660

A professional membership organization that works toward improving the quality of education for children with disabilities. Holds annual conference. Regular membership, $55.00. CEC's Division for the Visually Handicapped publishes its own newsletter four times per year. Division dues, $10.00.

Council of Citizens with Low Vision, International (CCLVI)
600 North Alabama Street
Tower 2, #2102
Indianapolis, IN 46204
(800) 733-2258

Provides support, education, and advocacy. Publishes "CCLVI News," a quarterly newsletter available in large print or on cassette. Membership, $5.00

Descriptive Video Service (DVS)
WGBH
125 Western Avenue
Boston, MA 02134
(617) 492-2777

This free national service makes television programs accessible to individuals who are visually impaired or blind. DVS is carried by many public stations in the United States. Publishes quarterly newsletter, "DVS Bulletin, available in large print, braille, or cassette. Free

Foundation for Glaucoma Research
490 Post Street, Suite 1042
San Francisco, CA 94102
(415) 986-3162

Supports research into the causes and treatment of glaucoma. Newsletter, "Gleams," free.

Glaucoma Foundation
310 East 14th Street
New York, NY 10003
(800) 832-3926   (212) 260-1000

Supports research into the causes and treatment of glaucoma.

Helen Keller National Center for Deaf-Blind Youths and Adults
111 Middle Neck Road
Sands Point, NY 11050
(516) 944-8900 (V/TDD)

Provides evaluation for rehabilitation through regional field offices throughout U.S. Publishes "National Center News," free.

Lighthouse National Center for Vision and Child Development
800 Second Avenue
New York, NY 10017
(800) 334-5497   (212) 355-2200   (212) 980-7832 (TDD)

Provides professional training, internships and student training; conducts applied and theoretical research; and develops educational materials for professionals and the general public.

National Association for Parents of Visually Impaired (NAPVI)
2180 Linway Drive
Beloit, WI 53511
(800) 562-6265

Promotes development of parent groups; provides information through conferences, publications, and quarterly newsletter, "Awareness." Local chapters in some states. Free information packet. Membership: families, $20.00; professionals, $25.00; agencies, $50.00.

National Association for Visually Handicapped (NAVH)
22 West 21st Street
New York, NY 10010
(212) 889-3141

Provides large print books on loan and for sale. Sells low vision and nonoptical aids. Free large print newsletters, "Seeing Clearly," for adults, and "In Focus," for youth.

National Center on Vision and Aging (NCVA)
800 Second Avenue
New York, NY 10017
(800) 334-5497   (212) 355-2200   (212) 980-7832 (TDD)

Provides information on vision problems faced by older people and how these problems can be treated. Sells community education material. Conducts conferences and training programs.

National Eye Institute (NEI)
Building 31, Room 6A32
Bethesda, MD 20892
(301) 496-5248

Conducts basic and clinical research. Produces public and professional education materials. Distributes free brochures on many eye diseases and conditions.

National Federation of the Blind (NFB)
1800 Johnson Street
Baltimore, MD 21230
(301) 659-9314

National membership organization with chapters in many states. Publishes the "Braille Monitor," a monthly magazine, available in print, braille, and on cassette. Subdivisions for parents of children who are visually impaired or blind; students; diabetics; and others.

National Library Service for the Blind and Physically Handicapped (NLS)
1291 Taylor Street, NW
Washington DC 20542
(800) 424-8567 or 8572

Provides services to all print-handicapped children and adults, including those who cannot hold a book or turn pages. Provides publications in braille; on cassette and flexible disc; and the machines to play them, free. Each state has at least one NLS regional library. Some NLS libraries distribute large print books.

Recording for the Blind (RFB)
20 Roszel Road
Princeton, NJ 08540
(800) 221-4792   In NJ, (609) 452-0606

Records educational materials for people who are legally blind or physically or perceptually handicapped. Requires certification of disability by a medical or educational professional. Charges a one-time registration fee of $25.00.

Resources for Rehabilitation
33 Bedford Street, Suite 19A
Lexington, MA 02173
(617) 862-6455

Provides information and training to professionals and the public about resources that help people with disabilities and chronic conditions, including vision loss. Publishes the "Living with Low Vision Series," described in "PUBLICATIONS AND TAPES" section below. Custom designed training programs available. Call for details.

RP Foundation Fighting Blindness
1401 Mt. Royal Avenue
Baltimore, MD 21217
(800) 638-2300   (301) 225-9400

Supports research, provides public and professional education materials, and publishes quarterly newsletter. Local chapters and information centers. Free publications including "Answers to Your Questions About Retinitis Pigmentosa and Other Retinal Degenerative Diseases."

VA Office of Technology Transfer
Prosthetics R&D Center
103 South Gay Street
Baltimore, MD 21202
(301) 962-1800

Sponsors rehabilitation research and development of assistive technology for visual impairment, blindness and other disabilities. Publishes "Journal of Rehabilitation Research and Development" (see "PUBLICATIONS AND TAPES" section below). The VA Rehabilitation Database includes abstracts of articles in the "Journal of Rehabilitation Research and Development." The database is available through CompuServe, a subscription computer network. Call Dori Grasso at the number listed above for help or for free introductory time on CompuServe.

VISION Foundation, Inc.
818 Mt. Auburn Street
Watertown, MA 02172
(617) 926-4232   In MA, (800) 852-3029

Information center for individuals with sight loss. Publishes VISION Resource List; VISION Resource Update, a bimonthly resource newsletter; and VISION VIEWS, an annual organization newsletter. Regular membership, $20.00; seniors, $10.00.

Business is Looking Up
by Barbara Aiello and Jeffrey Shulman
9385-C Gerwig Lane
Columbia, MD 21046
(800) 368-5437   (301) 290-9095

One of "The Kids on the Block" series, this book, with a character who has low vision, is written for children in grades two to five. $12.95

Children's Braille Book Club
National Braille Press
88 St. Stephen Street
Boston, MA 02115
(617) 266-6160

Braille pages are inserted into standard print children's books. Free membership provides monthly notices with no obligation to buy; $100.00 annual subscription automatically provides one print-braille book per month.

Dialogue
Blindskills, Inc.
Box 5181
Salem, OR 97304
(503) 581-4224

Quarterly magazine with information on technology and other resources, special information on child rearing for blind parents, and an announcements section. Published in braille, large print, and 4-track cassette (playable on a National Library Service Talking Book Cassette Player). $20.00

The First Steps: How To Help People Who Are Losing Their Sight
Peninsula Center for the Blind
4151 Middlefield Road
Palo Alto, CA 94303
(415) 858-0202

A booklet written to answer some of the initial questions and discuss some of the immediate reactions people have when blindness first occurs in a family. $8.25

If Blindness Strikes: Don't Strike Out
by Margaret Smith
Charles C. Thomas, Springfield, IL

Written by a visually impaired rehabilitation counselor, this book describes many adaptations and strategies for living with vision loss. $36.25. Cassette version may be purchased from Readings for the Blind, 29451 Greenfield Road, Suite 118, Southfield, MI 48076. 2-track ($13.50) or 4-track ($7.50) Also available on 4-track cassette on loan from the National Library Service for the Blind and Physically Handicapped through local regional libraries, RC 21060. (800) 484-8567 or 8572

Journal of Rehabilitation Research and Development (JRRD)
Office of Technology Transfer
VA Prosthetics R&D Center
103 South Gay Street
Baltimore, MD 21202

A quarterly publication of scientific and engineering articles including those related to sensory aids and gerontology. Includes abstracts of literature, book reviews, and calendar of events. For sale by U.S. Superintendent of Documents, Government Printing Office, Washington DC 20402

Journal of Visual Impairment and Blindness (JVIB)
American Foundation for the Blind
15 West 16th Street
New York, NY 10011
(800) 232-5463   (212) 620-2000

Publishes original research in the field of visual impairment and blindness. Includes information on legislation affecting individuals who are visually impaired or blind and a calendar of events. Ten issues a year, $45.00

Just Enough to Know Better
by Eileen Curran
National Braille Press
88 St. Stephen Street
Boston, MA 02115
(617) 266-6160

This self paced workbook teaches beginning braille skills to sighted parents. $12.50

Lifeprints
Blindskills, Inc.
Box 5181
Salem, OR 97304
(503) 581-4224

Magazine with focus on careers and life skills of youth and adults who are visually impaired or blind. Large print, cassette, or braille. $15.00

Living with Low Vision Series
Resources for Rehabilitation
33 Bedford Street, Suite 19A
Lexington, MA 02173
(617) 862-6455

"LARGE PRINT Publications Designed for Distribution by Professionals to People with Vision Loss" Titles include "Living with Low Vision," "How to Keep Reading with Vision Loss," "Aids for Everyday Living with Vision Loss," and disease specific titles. (See order form opposite inside back cover for complete list of titles and prices.)

"Living with Low Vision: A Resource Guide for People with Sight Loss"
A comprehensive directory that helps people with sight loss locate services they need to remain independent. Describes products that enable people to keep reading, working, and carrying out their daily activities. Large print. $35.00 plus $5.00 shipping and handling

"Providing Services for People with Vision Loss: A Multidisciplinary Perspective"
Susan L. Greenblatt (ed.)

Volume 1
Written by ophthalmologists and rehabilitation professionals, this book discusses the need to provide coordinated care for people with vision loss. Chapters include Vision Loss: A Patient's Perspective; Operating a Low Vision Aids Service; Vision Loss: An Ophthalmologist's Perspective; The Need for Coordinated Care; Making Referrals for Rehabilitation Services; Mental Health Services: The Missing Link; Self-Help Groups for People with Sight Loss; and Aids and Techniques that Help People with Vision Loss plus a Glossary. Also available on cassette. $19.95 plus $3.00 shipping and handling

Volume 2
Written by physicians, special educators, counselors, and rehabilitation professionals, this book includes chapters on What People with Vision Loss Need to Know; The Special Needs of Individuals with Diabetes and Vision Loss; Older Adults with Vision and Hearing Losses; Providing Services to Visually Impaired Elders in Long Term Care Facilities; Children with Vision Loss; and The Role of the Family, $24.95 plus $3.00 shipping and handling

"Rehabilitation Resource Manual: VISION"
A professional desk reference that includes information on the rehabilitation process for individuals with vision loss; how to make referrals; a bibliography; and hundreds of nationwide referral sources. Chapters on services and products for special population groups and by eye conditions and diseases. $39.95 plus $5.00 shipping and handling

Low Vision: What You Can Do To Preserve - And Even Enhance - Your Usable Sight
by Helen Neal
Simon and Schuster, New York, NY

Describes the health professionals, programs, optical aids, and techniques that are a part of low vision services. Lists sources of catalogues, products, services and support groups. $8.95

Making Life More Livable
by Irving R. Dickman
American Foundation for the Blind
15 West 16th Street
New York, NY 10011
(800) 232-5463   (212) 620-2000

Offers simple adaptations to make the home safer for those with vision impairment. $9.95 plus $3.00 shipping and handling. Also available on 4-track cassette on loan through the National Library Service for the Blind and Physically Handicapped through local regional libraries, RC 22319. (800) 424-8567 or 8572

Meeting the Needs of Employees with Disabilities
Resources for Rehabilitation
33 Bedford Street, Suite 19A
Lexington, MA 02173
(617) 862-6455

Provides information to help people with disabilities retain or obtain employment. Information on government programs, environmental adaptations, and the transition from school to work are included. Chapters on mobility, vision, and hearing and speech impairments include information on organizations, products, and services that enable employers to accommodate the needs of employees with disabilities. $42.95 plus $5.00 shipping and handling

Pathways to Independence: Orientation and Mobility Skills for Your Infant and Toddler
National Center for Vision and Child Development
800 Second Avenue
New York, NY 10017
(800) 334-5497   (212) 355-2200

Discusses basic orientation and mobility skills and suggests games and activities for the child with vision loss. $2.50

Questions Kids Ask About Blindness
National Federation of the Blind (NFB)
1800 Johnson Street
Baltimore, MD 21230
(301) 659-9314

Answers general questions about blindness, braille, canes, guide dogs, and the abilities of individuals who are visually impaired or blind. Describes a typical day in the life of a blind sixth grader attending public school. $3.50

Resources for Elders with Disabilities
Resources for Rehabilitation
33 Bedford Street, Suite 19A
Lexington, MA 02173
(617) 862-6455

A large print resource directory that describes services and products that help elders with disabilities to function independently. Includes chapters on vision loss, hearing loss, stroke, arthritis, diabetes, and osteoporosis. $39.95 plus $5.00 shipping and handling

Seedlings
PO Box 2395
Livonia, MI 48151-0395
(313) 427-8552

Publishes inexpensive children's storybooks in braille. Free catalogue.

Some Answers About Glaucoma
National Glaucoma Research
15825 Shady Grove Road, Suite 140
Rockville, MD 20850
(800) 227-7998

Describes the major types of glaucoma, risk factors, diagnosis and treatment, and lists helpful references, toll-free numbers, and organizations. Large print. Free

TRAVEL TALES - A Mobility Storybook
Mostly Mobility
R.D. #1, Box 1448-A
Bethel, PA 19507

Designed to teach mobility to children in preschool through third grade, this book may be used by parents of children who are visually impaired or blind, classroom teachers, special education teachers, as well as orientation and mobility teachers. $22.00

<u>The Visually Handicapped Child in Your Classroom</u>
by Elizabeth K. Chapman and Juliet M. Stone
Brookes Publishing Company
PO Box 10624
Baltimore, MD 21285-9945
(800) 638-3775

Provides practical suggestions for educators on integrating children who are visually impaired or blind into the classroom. $21.50

Listed below are catalogues that specialize in devices for people who are visually impaired or blind. Unless otherwise noted, catalogues are free.

Exceptional Teaching Aids
20102 Woodbine Avenue
Castro Valley, CA 94546
(415) 582-4859

Braille and low vision aids; adaptive computer software; art, science, and mathematical aids.

Independent Living Aids, Inc.
27 East Mall
Plainview, NY 11803
(800) 537-2118   (516) 752-8080

LS&S Group Inc. Catalogue
PO Box 673
Northbrook, IL 60065
(800) 468-4789   In IL, (708) 498-9777

Print copy, free; cassette, $3.00, applied to first purchase.

Maxi-Vision
42 Executive Boulevard
PO Box 3209
Farmingdale, NY 11735
(800) 522-6294   (516) 752-0521

Products for People with Vision Problems
American Foundation for the Blind
15 West 16th Street
New York, NY 10011
(800) 232-5463   (212) 620-2000

Catalogue available in standard print and braille.

Science Products
Box A
Southeastern, PA 19399
(800) 822-7400

Specially adapted scientific and technical instruments plus the standard variety of aids.

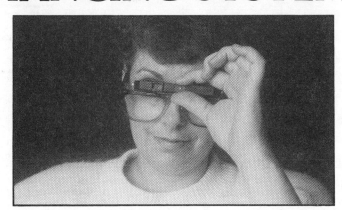
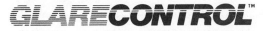

203

Low-Vision Word Processor:
☞ just $295!

In this actual PC screen, the text is smooth--not blocky.

- *Eye Relief* is an award-winning Word Processing program for Low-Vision users. It lets the Low-Vision user do word processing with high-quality screen fonts and complete control over on-screen spacing. *Eye Relief* runs on any PC that has 512K of RAM and a graphics screen. (CGA, EGA, VGA, or Hercules.)

- *Eye Relief* screen fonts can be 1,2,3,4 or 5x normal size--up to 1.4" high on a standard PC screen! As you type and edit, your text will appear in large type--as will on-screen help, pull-down menus, and other messages. Even the *User Guide* is set in 18-point Large Type!

- *Eye Relief* lets you create, edit, and print standard ASCII text files. (This insures compatibility with other word processors, as files created by *Eye Relief* may be loaded easily into WordPerfect, Microsoft Word, and other word processors.)

- Editing functions include Insert, Delete, Cut, Paste, Copy, Find and Replace. Text *wordwraps* at the edge of the screen, so you always see a continuous stream of text. (No need for horizontal scrolling!)

Note: The text shown above would be **TWICE** as large on a standard 14" PC screen.

If you have macular degeneration, just increase the space between the lines! ◀

Eye Relief is a trademark of SkiSoft Publishing Corporation.

- It prints normal-sized text on any printer, using any margins, headers, footers, and page numbers. It can print 18-point Type on a Laserjet or Postscript printer.

Eye Relief is a product of SkiSoft Publishing Corporation
1644 Massachusetts Ave. Suite 79
Lexington, MA 02173

617-863-1876 Fax: 617-861-0086

Order now--or request a demo!

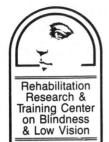
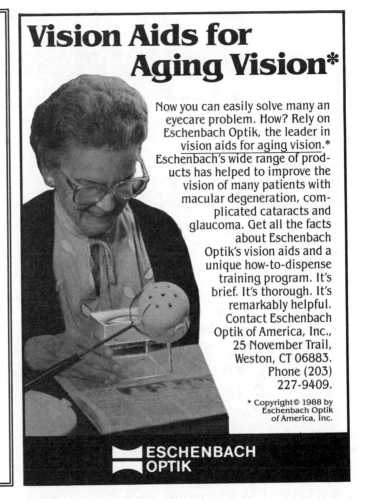

APPENDIX A

MAIN OFFICES OF STATE VOCATIONAL REHABILITATION AGENCIES

To learn the address of the state agency nearest you, contact the main office listed below or the information operator for the state government.

Alabama
Rehabilitation Services
Department of Education
Montgomery, AL 36111
(205) 281-8780
(205) 281-8780, ext. 249 (TDD)

Alaska
Office of Vocational Rehabilitation
PO Box F MS 0581
Juneau, AK 99811
(907) 465-2814
(907) 465-2440 (TDD)

Arizona
Rehabilitation Services Administration
1300 West Washington
Phoenix, AZ 85007
(602) 542-3323 (V/TDD)
In AZ, (800) 352-8161

Arkansas
Division of Rehabilitation Services
720 West Third Street
Little Rock, AR 72201
(501) 324-9106

California
Department of Rehabilitation
830 K Street Mall
Sacramento, CA 95814
(916) 445-3971

Colorado
Rehabilitation Services
1575 Sherman, 4th floor
Denver, CO 80203-1714
(303) 866-5196
(303) 866-3258 (TDD)

Connecticut
Division of Rehabilitation Services
10 Griffin Road
North Windsor, CT 06095
(203) 298-2000 (V/TDD)
In CT, (800) 537-2549

Delaware
Department of Health and Social Services
1901 North Dupont Highway, Biggs Building
Newcastle, DE 19720
(302) 421-6748

District of Columbia
Rehabilitation Services Administration
1120 G Street NW, 6th Floor
Washington, DC 20005
(202) 727-8620

Florida
Division of Vocational Rehabilitation
1709A Mahan Drive
Tallahassee, FL 32399-0696
(904) 488-6210
(904) 488-2867 (TDD)

Georgia
Division of Rehabilitation Services
878 Peachtree Street, Room 706
Atlanta, GA 30309
(404) 894-6670 (V/TDD)

Hawaii
Department of Human Services
1901 Bachelot Street
Honolulu, HI 96817
(800) 548-6367

Idaho
Division of Vocational Rehabilitation
650 West State Street
Boise, ID 83702
(208) 334-3390 (V/TDD)

Illinois
Illinois Department of Rehabilitation
Services
623 East Adams Street
PO Box 19429
Springfield, IL 62794-9429
(217) 782-2093
(217) 782-5734 (TDD)

Indiana
Department of Human Resources
251 North Illinois Street
PO Box 7083
Indianapolis, IN 46207-7083
(317) 232-1147

Iowa
Division of Vocational Rehabilitation
Services
510 East Twelfth Street
Des Moines, IA 50309
(515) 281-4311
In IA, (800) 532-1486
(515) 281-6755 (TDD)

Kansas
Rehabilitation Services
Biddle Building, 1st Floor
300 SW Oakley Street
Topeka, KS 66606
(913) 296-3911
In KS, (800) 432-2326
(913) 296-7029 (TDD)

Kentucky
Office of Vocational Rehabilitation
Capital Plaza Tower, 9th floor
500 Mero Street
Frankfort, KY 40601
(502) 564-4440
In KY (800) 372-7172
(502) 564-6817 (TDD)

Louisiana
Department of Social Services
Rehabilitation Services
1755 Florida Boulevard
PO Box 94371
Baton Rouge, LA 70804-9371
(504) 342-2285
(504) 342-2266 (TDD)

Maine
Bureau of Rehabilitation
35 Anthony Avenue
Augusta, ME 04333-0011
(207) 626-5300
(207) 626-5322

Maryland
Division of Vocational Rehabilitation
2301 Argonne Drive
Baltimore, MD 21218-1696
(301) 554-3276
(301) 554-3277 (TDD)

Massachusetts
Massachusetts Rehabilitation Commission
Fort Point Place
27-43 Wormwood Street
Boston, MA 02110
(617) 727-2183
In MA, (800) 442-1171
(617) 727-9063 (TDD)

Michigan
Rehabilitation Services
608 West Allegan, PO Box 30010
Lansing, MI 48909
(517) 373-3391
In MI, (800) 292-5896
(517) 373-3980 (V/TDD)

Minnesota
Division of Rehabilitation Services
390 North Robert
St. Paul, MN 55101
(612) 296-5616
In MN, (800) 328-9095
(612) 296-3900 (TDD)

Mississippi
Vocational Rehabilitation
PO Box 1698
Jackson, MS 39215
(601) 354-6677
In MS, (800) 443-1000
(601) 354-6830 (TDD)

Missouri
Division of Vocational Rehabilitation
201 East McCarty Street
Jefferson City, MO 65101
(314) 751-3251
(314) 751-0881 (TDD)

Montana
Department of Social and Rehabilitation
Services
111 Sanders Street, PO Box 4210
Helena, MT 59604-4210
(406) 444-2590 (V/TDD)

Nebraska
Division of Rehabilitation Services
301 Centennial Mall South, 6th floor
PO Box 94987
Lincoln, NE 68509-4987
(402) 471-3652 (V/TDD)

Nevada
Rehabilitation Services
505 East King, Room 502
Carson City, NV 89710
(702) 687-4440 (V/TDD)

New Hampshire
Division of Vocational Rehabilitation
78 Regional Drive, Building 2
Concord, NH 03301
(603) 271-3471
In NH, (800) 992-3312 (TDD)

New Jersey
Labor Building, 6th floor
CN 398
Trenton, NJ 08625
(609) 292-5987
(609) 292-2919 (TDD)

New Mexico
Division of Vocational Rehabilitation
604 West San Mateo Drive
Santa Fe, NM 87503
(505) 827-3511
In NM, (800) 235-5387
(505) 827-3510 (TDD)

New York
Office of Vocational and Educational
Services for Individuals with Disabilities
One Commerce Plaza, Room 1606
Albany, NY 12234
(518) 474-2714
In NY, (800) 222-5627
(518) 473-9333 (TDD)

North Carolina
Division of Vocational Rehabilitation
Services
805 Ruggles Drive
PO Box 26053
Raleigh, NC 27611
(919) 733-3364
(919) 733-5924 (TDD)

North Dakota
Office of Vocational Rehabilitation
State Capitol, Judicial Wing
600 East Boulevard Avenue
Bismarck, ND 58505-0250
(701) 224-2907
In ND, (800) 472-2622
(701) 224-2699 (TDD)

Ohio
Rehabilitation Services Commission
400 East Campus View Boulevard
Columbus, OH 43235-4604
(614) 438-1200
In OH, (800) 282-4536
(614) 438-1391 (TDD)

Oklahoma
Rehabilitation Services
2409 North Kelley, 4th Floor Annex
PO Box 25352
Oklahoma City, OK 73125
(405) 424-4311
(405) 424-2794 (TDD)

Oregon
Rehabilitation Services
2045 Silverton Road, NE
Salem, OR 97310
(503) 378-3830 (V/TDD)

Pennsylvania
Office of Vocational Rehabilitation
7th and Forster Street
Harrisburg, PA 17120
(717) 787-4256
In PA, (800) 442-6351
(717) 783-8917 (TDD)

Puerto Rico
Vocational Rehabilitation Program
Box 1118
Hato Rey, PR 00919
(809) 725-1792

Rhode Island
Department of Vocational Rehabilitation
40 Fountain Street
Providence, RI 02903
(401) 421-7005
In RI, (800) 752-8088
(401) 421-7016 (TDD)

South Carolina
Vocational Rehabilitation Department
1330 Boston Avenue
West Columbia, SC 29201
(803) 822-5319 (V/TDD)

South Dakota
Division of Rehabilitation Services
700 Governors Drive
Pierre, SD 57501-2291
(605) 773-3195
(605) 773-4544 (TDD)

Tennessee
Division of Rehabilitation Services
400 Deaderick Street, 15th floor
Nashville, TN 37248-0060
(615) 741-2019

Texas
Rehabilitation Commission
4900 North Lamar Boulevard
Austin, TX 78751-2316
(512) 483-4000
(512) 483-4884 (TDD)

Utah
Office of Rehabilitation
250 East 500 South
Salt Lake City, UT 84111
(801) 538-7522
In UT, (800) 662-9080 (TDD)

Vermont
Vocational Rehabilitation Division
Osgood Building
103 South Main Street
Waterbury, VT 05671-2301
(802) 241-2186 (V/TDD)

Virginia
Department Rehabilitative Services
4901 Fitzhugh Avenue
Richmond, VA 23230
(804) 367-0316
In VA, (800) 552-5019
(804) 367-0315 (TDD)

Washington
Vocational Rehabilitation Services
Office Building 2, OB-21C
Olympia, WA 98504
(206) 753-0293
In WA, (800) 637-5627 (V/TDD)

West Virginia
Division of Rehabilitation Services
PO Box 1004
Institute, WV 25305
(304) 766-4600
(304) 766-4969(TDD)

Wisconsin
Division of Vocational Rehabilitation
1 West Wilson Street
PO Box 7852
Madison, WI 53707
(608) 266-1281
(608) 266-9599 (TDD)

Wyoming
Division of Rehabilitation Services
1100 Herschler Building
Cheyenne, WY 82002
(307) 777-7389 (V/TDD)

INDEX TO ORGANIZATIONS

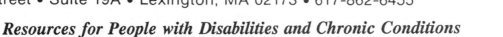

RESOURCES for REHABILITATION

33 Bedford Street • Suite 19A • Lexington, MA 02173 • 617-862-6455

Resources for People with Disabilities and Chronic Conditions

comprehensive resource directory with chapters on spinal cord injuries, low back pain, diabetes, multiple sclerosis, hearing and speech impairments, vision impairment and blindness, and epilepsy. Includes information about the disease or condition; psychological aspects of the condition; professional services providers; environmental adaptations; assistive devices; and descriptions of organizations, publications, and products. Special information for children is also included. ISBN 0-929718-06-2 $44.95

Meeting the Needs of Employees with Disabilities

This book provides employers and counselors with the information they need to help people with disabilities retain or obtain employment. Information on government programs and laws, supported employment, training programs, environmental adaptations, and the transition from school to work are included. Chapters on mobility, vision, and hearing and speech impairments include information on organizations, products, and services that enable employers to accommodate the needs of employees with disabilities. ISBN 0-929718-08-9 $42.95

Resources for Elders with Disabilities

Printed in **18 point bold** type, this book includes information on the diseases that cause common disabilities, the major rehabilitation networks, self-help groups, and legislation that affects people with disabilities. Chapters on hearing loss, vision loss, diabetes, arthritis, osteoporosis, and stroke describe assistive devices, organizations, and publications that help people with these conditions. 1990 ISBN 0-929718-03-8 $39.95

Living with Low Vision: A Resource Guide for People with Sight Loss

LARGE PRINT (**18 point bold type**) comprehensive directory that helps people with sight loss locate the services, products, and publications that they need to keep reading, working, and enjoying life. Chapters for children, elders, and people with both hearing and vision loss plus self-help groups, how to keep working with vision loss, and making everyday living easier. Second edition. 1990 ISBN 0-929718-04-6 $35.00

Rehabilitation Resource Manual: VISION

desk reference that enables professionals to make effective referrals. Includes information on understanding the responses to vision loss; breaking the news of irreversible vision loss; guidelines on starting self-help groups; information on professional research and service organizations; plus chapters on optical and nonoptical aids; for special populations; and by eye condition/disease. Third edition. 1990 ISBN 0-929718-05-4 $39.95

Providing Services for People with Vision Loss: A Multidisciplinary Perspective

Susan L. Greenblatt, Editor

This book discusses how various professionals can work together to provide coordinated care for people with vision loss. Chapters include Vision Loss: A Patient's Perspective; Operating a Low Vision Aids Service; Vision Loss: An Ophthalmologist's Perspective;   The Need for Coordinated Care;   Making Referrals for Rehabilitation Services; Mental Health Services: The Missing Link; Self-Help Groups for People with Sight Loss; and Aids and Techniques that Help People with Vision Loss plus a Glossary. Also available on cassette. 1989
ISBN 0-929718-02-X $19.95

LARGE PRINT PUBLICATIONS

Designed for distribution by professionals to people with disabilities and chronic conditions
Printed in 18 point bold type, these very special publications include information on each condition, rehabilitation services and professionals, products, and resources that help people with disabilities and chronic conditions to live independently. Titles include **Living with Hearing Loss, Living with Arthritis, After a Stroke, Living with Diabetes, Living with Low Vision, How to Keep Reading with Vision Loss,** and **Aging and Vision Loss.** Printed on ivory paper with black ink for maximum contrast. 8 1/2" by 11"

Discounts available on purchases of 10 or more copies of any book title.

RESOURCES for REHABILITATION

33 Bedford Street • Suite 19A • Lexington, MA 02173 • 617-862-6455

Our Federal Employer Identification Number is 04-2975-007

NAME _____

ORGANIZATION _____

ADDRESS _____

PHONE _____

[ ] Check or signed institutional purchase order enclosed for full amount of order. Purchase ord(
accepted from government agencies, hospitals, and universities <u>only</u>.

[ ]Mastercard/VISA Card number: _____

Expiration date:_____ Signature: _____

ALL ORDERS OF $50.00 OR LESS <u>MUST</u> BE PREPAID.

TITLE	QUANTITY		PRICE	TOTAL
Resources for people with disabilities and chronic conditions	____	X	$44.95	_____
Meeting the needs of employees with disabilities	____	X	42.95	_____
Resources for elders with disabilities	____	X	39.95	_____
Living with low vision: A resource guide	____	X	35.00	_____
Rehabilitation resource manual: VISION	____	X	39.95	_____
Providing services for people with vision loss	____	X	19.95	_____

<u>MINIMUM PURCHASE OF 25 COPIES PER TITLE FOR THE FOLLOWING PUBLICATIONS</u>
Call for discount on purchases of 100 or more copies of any single title.

Living with arthritis	____	X	2.00	_____
Living with hearing loss	____	X	2.00	_____
After a stroke	____	X	2.00	_____
Living with diabetes	____	X	2.00	_____
Living with low vision	____	X	2.00	_____
How to keep reading with vision loss	____	X	1.75	_____
Living with diabetic retinopathy	____	X	1.75	_____
Aging and vision loss	____	X	1.25	_____
Living with age-related macular degeneration	____	X	1.00	_____
Aids for everyday living with vision loss	____	X	1.25	_____
High tech aids for people with vision loss	____	X	1.75	_____

SUB - TOTAL
_____

SHIPPING & HANDLING: $25.00 or less, add $3.00; $25.01 to 50.00, add $5.00;
$50.01 to 100.00, add $7.00; add $2.00 for each additional $100.00 or fraction
of $100.00. For shipping to Canada, add $2.00 to shipping & handling charges.
Foreign orders must be prepaid in US currency. Please write for shipping charges.

TOTAL
$_____

Prices are subject to change.